**This book**
will help if you have back aches, if you are not sick in the full
sense of the word, but are plagued by pain in the small of the
back, neck, or in the muscles between the shoulder blades. It
also tells you what to do if you have just suffered a real medical
problem such as disc surgery, a sciatic attack or an acute attack
of lumbago.

It will also help you to find out what you can still expect from
your back, when you will be able to participate in sports again,
lift and carry, when you will be able to return to work or
household duties.

Renate Zauner, physical therapist of twenty years experience,
and Professor Albert Göb, head of the orthopedic department of
the University Clinic of Munich, answer all questions pertaining
to back pain. Back pains and their causes are fully and
understandably explained. The aim of this book is to offer you
therapeutic aid and simple exercises that will help you feel
better.

**Renate Zauner**
Born 1925 in Gross-Rosenburg near Magdeburg, Renate Zauner
grew up in East Prussia, Karlsruhe and Goettingen. Ten
semesters of medical school in Goettingen were interrupted by
marriage and the birth of two sons. She then studied to become
a licensed physical therapist in Goettingen. Since 1968, she has
written and published several popular medical books. Since
1961, Mrs. Zauner has lived in Munich with her family where
she has her own physical therapy practice.

**Prof. Albert Göb, M.D.**
Professor Göb was born in 1918. He studied medicine in Munich
and taught orthopedic medicine from 1955 to 1960 at the State
Physiotherapy School of Munich. In 1956, Prof. Göb founded
the Spastic Center of Munich, which he still heads. He is also
head of orthopedics at the Polyclinic of the University of
Munich.

Renate Zauner

# Speaking of:
# Back-
# Aches

Advice and help on disc problems,
wear and tear of the spinal column,
muscle spasm, sciatica, headaches
and migraines

With 70 Medical Gymnastic Exercises

Introduction: Prof. Albert Göb, M.D.

Translated by Martha Humphreys

*Consolidated Book Publishers*

NEW YORK • CHICAGO

Library of Congress Catalog Card Number: 78-72877
ISBN: 0-8326-2233-8

Originally published in German under the title *Sprechstunde:
Rückenschmerzen,* copyright © 1978 by Gräfe und Unzer Verlag,
München.

# Contents

# Introduction

Almost 50% of all people who must abandon active work do so
because of a significant loss of mobility of the back. They must
live with occasional or constant pain resulting from worn discs
or spondylitis (poker spine).

*Backaches
are third in
frequency*

Backaches rank third among the diseases characteristic of
highly industrialized societies, following heart-circulatory diseases and cancer. Most areas of contemporary medicine make
extensive use of preventive measures in the form of information
and frequent checkups, but changes in the back are detected
only when they produce pain.

Precautions against back illnesses require an understanding of
the relationships within the organism's biological processes and
a systematic method of learning to move properly. For this
purpose, the observations and experiences of a physiotherapist
can be very helpful.

What is new in this book is that changes in the back are not
judged solely from an orthopedic point of view. Diseases
resulting from changes—muscular strain, postural deterioration,
and manifestations of wear and tear—are considered from the
standpoint of the functional unity of the entire body and mind
and are thereby included among psychosomatic manifestions of
disease.

*Patients
want to be
informed*

Patients have a great need to know and understand what
causes backaches. Persons who are in constant pain consider it
important to know what causes their pain, what changes have
taken place in their backs and what they can still expect from

7

their backs after disc surgery or after an attack of sciatica or lumbago.

Physiotherapy provides supplementary treatment as well as continuation of a doctor's therapy. Patients often must be released from the hospital before they are "completely cured" because of a shortage of hospital beds and the necessity of keeping costs down. Consequently, the patient must be ambulatory during recovery, and professional help is mandatory during this period. Regardless of whether the patient is being treated by a neurologist, surgeon, orthopedist or internist, often only physiotherapy can provide the patient with the necessary physical and emotional assistance for resuming a normal life.

By providing detailed, comprehensible answers to questions repeatedly posed by every patient, this book fills a gap. It also provides guidance in the prevention of back problems. It offers practical help that enables every patient to work actively toward his own recovery.

*Cooperation between doctor and physiotherapist*

The book also shows for the first time the importance of coordinating medical and physiotherapeutic treatment. In addition, the patient is included in discussing which form of therapy is most suitable and effective, thereby complying with the legitimate right of every patient to full and comprehensible information.

The extensive use of physiotherapy is still relatively recent, having achieved its present significance only within the last 25 years. It is important for the rehabilitation of patients being treated by orthopedics and by surgery. As an experienced teacher at the Munich School of Physiotherapy, it is particularly important to me that the many possibilities of physical therapy be fully used.

*Prof. Göb, M.D.*

# 1. The Functional Unity of the Back

Our highly civilized world offers many conveniences, particularly in the area of technology; and it has made life much easier than in former times. Our standard of living, however, exacts a high price that is paid by many people in the form of pain, latent impairment to their health, and premature wear and tear on their bodies. These sufferings are caused not only by physical overexertion; they are often the result of emotional pressure, overexertion, and other stress situations.

One of the most important areas affected by such various forms of exertion is the back. Despite its seemingly sturdy bony supporting apparatus and its compact muscular structure, it is very suspectible to all forms of physical and psychological overexertion and always reacts in the same manner—with pain.

Back pains result from early wear and tear of the discs, from irregular muscle function due to poor posture, or from cramps of the musculature, regardless of whether these are caused by physical or emotional overexertion.

*Biological unity of body and mind*
Pathological changes in the area of the back and the resulting discomforts must therefore be considered and evaluated from other than a strictly orthopedic point of view. Since body and mind represent a functional and biological unity, many of these complaints can be considered psychosomatic manifestations of disease and, from this perspective, can to a large extent be explained.

The purpose of this book is to provide answers to all manner of responses—including psychosomatic responses to back pain,

9

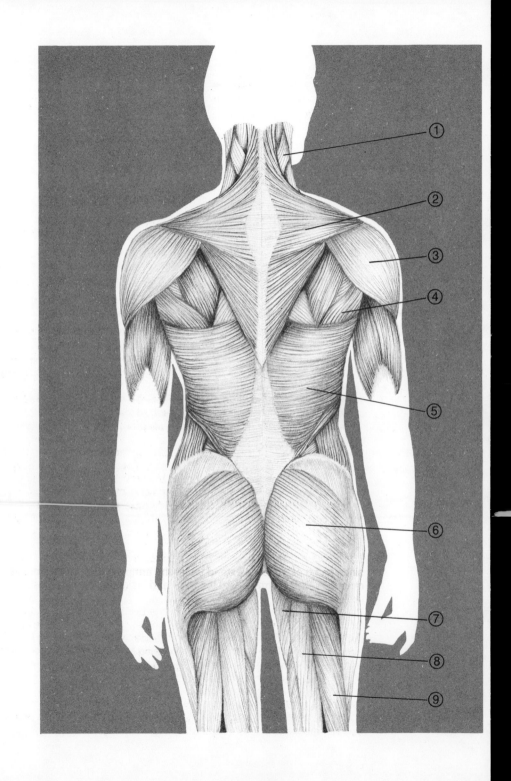

① 

② 

③ 

④ 

⑤ 

⑥ 

⑦ 

⑧ 

⑨

questions concerning all these reactions, manifestations of detrition, and occasional or constant back pain. It also explains the relationship between back strain, changes in the back, and back pain.

# The Layman's Right to Information

The questions dealt with here are those that arise most often during my practice. They are asked repeatedly by patients during physical therapy treatments or massages and reveal the helplessness with which they regard their problems. The questions also reveal the extent of the patients' need for enlightenment, an understanding of the context of the problem, and a need also to participate actively in regaining health and in completely resuming productive lives.

A patient's lack of knowledge about his own illness leads to

*Important questions asked by patients*

---

*The surfaces of the back musculature in which basically the processes occur that may result in back pain.*

**1.** *musculus splenius capitis* (strap muscle)—main function: if both sides of the spine contract simultaneously, it pulls the head into the neck; if only one side contracts, the head turns in the direction of the side that is contracted.

**2.** *musculus trapezius* (trapezius muscle), formerly called cowl muscle. Main function: to lift, lower, and pull back the shoulders; to carry weight.

**3.** *musculus deltoideus* (deltoid muscle) is the essential arm-lifter. It also assists in twisting the arm and in moving the arm forward and backward, especially if the arm is already raised to a 60° angle.

**4.** *musculus teres major* (large round muscle)—main function: to turn the arm toward the inside, pull it toward the back, and lower it from a raised position.

**5.** *musculus latissimus dorsi* (the broad back muscle)—main function: since some of its fibers extend under the armpit to the upper arm, this muscle pulls the arm toward the back and inside; it is the apron string muscle.

**6.** *musculus glutaeus maximus* (the large buttocks muscle)—main function: to stretch in the hips, to move the thigh of the leg that is not taking the weight toward the rear, to stabilize the weight-bearing leg, making it possible to pull the leg not bearing the weight toward the rear. Also used in climbing mountains or going up stairs.

**7.** *musculus semimembranaceus* (the half skin muscle).

**8.** *musculus semitendineus* (the half tendon muscle).

**9.** *musculus biceps femoris* (the two-headed thigh muscle).

The last three muscles work together. They stretch in the hips and bend in the knee.

11

doubts about himself and his strength, destroys his trust in the functional ability of his own organism, and impedes cooperation between doctor and patient. This is particularly true of patients who have had a serious illness—a serious attack of sciatica, an acute lumbago attack, or a disc problem treated by surgery. They ask such questions as: "Will I be allowed to lift and carry objects again? Drive a car? Participate in sports? Will my back be able to sustain the burden of occupational and household duties?" Lack of knowledge is also a handicap for persons with everyday back problems, for persons who are not actually ill but who repeatedly have complaints.

Many persons may experience backache during work—the secretary at the typewriter, the housewife doing housework, the factory worker at a machine, the manager sitting at a desk. They experience back pain when bending, standing, or sitting for a long time, or during a long car drive. They come to me with such diagnoses as cervical vertebral column syndrome, myogelosis, postural anomalies, sciatic syndrome. They have no idea what these words mean, because they do not know or understand the context of changes that have occurred in their spinal columns or discs.

Many know the terms, the medical jargon that they have heard for years, but they are nonetheless unable to break out of the vicious cycle of physical and emotional stress; their back muscles cramp again and again and cause back pain. Regardless of social status or the strenuousness of their work or physical exertion, they suffer discomfort without knowing why or what it means. Most of these patients are able to work, although some

*When is a person healthy again?*

consider themselves really sick. More difficult questions for them are: "When is a person really well again? What is considered healthy about a spinal column with worn-out discs?

Lumbago has an acute beginning; it is the real start of a disease, yet its termination is merely a tapering-off process, because its cause, a worn-out disc, is still present. It is necessary to learn to live with it by treating it properly and by moving sensibly, because its dependable response to abuse and exertion is always heightened tensing of the muscles, resulting in cramps and finally in pain. Each back has its specific strain

---

*The human spinal column.* The illustration shows its physiological function. Since it connects separate sections of the body with one another, changes in this area affect the whole organism.

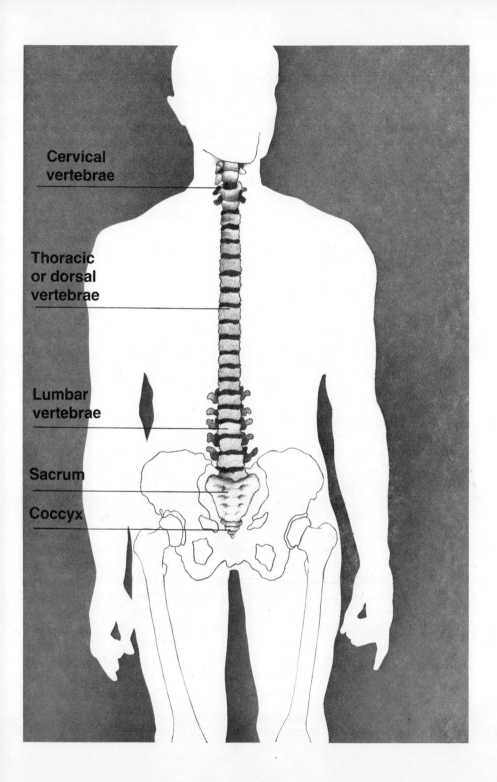

Cervical
vertebrae

Thoracic
or dorsal
vertebrae

Lumbar
vertebrae

Sacrum

Coccyx

tolerance. If it is not exceeded and if the person can correctly estimate the amount his back will tolerate, it is possible to live with worn discs. A manifestation of wear is not in itself a disease and does not necessarily cause pain. It is important, however, to know which changes take place in the spinal column over the years and how the musculature of the back responds to physical and emotional strain. The patient should also learn what he himself can do toward the maintenance of a healthy back, both in terms of unburdening it and helping it function.

# The Relationship between Therapist and Patient

A doctor's first concern must be for the acutely ill. After removing a disc, the surgeon loses contact with the patient if the follow-up care in the hospital is without complications, simply because the next emergency awaits him. There is too little time for the patient's questions. Many problems arise only later because of overexertion at work, at home, or in sports activities. The patient, having become more aware of certain painful conditions, attempts to interpret them. What does a feeling of pressure above the sacral area mean, for example? Or the feeling of a pull in the calf, of a stabbing pain between the shoulder blades? When does the feeling of numbness in the leg after disc surgery cease? The family physician is often overwhelmed by these seemingly irrelevant questions even though each question concerns important bodily changes. Often considerations concerning the family, job, or some special situation are factors contributing to pain. And the process of interpreting the symptoms and of answering the patient's many perfectly valid questions requires more time than the doctor, even with the best intentions, can spare. The situation is also complicated by the fact that the patient often does not realize that his backache is caused by his relationship with a co-worker rather than by a desk that is allegedly too low. A young woman's repeated sciatic attacks may not be due to a cold or an irritated nerve but to greater muscle tension prior to her divorce hearing.

For all of these reasons, physiotherapy can provide a vitally important contribution, for it offers a combination of guided

manual therapy and physical rehabilitation plus the time and
patience lacking in medical practice.

*Types of
massage
therapy*

This particular form of therapeutic treatment requires familiarity, a friendship without ties, but one that grows in time. It
offers the person a certain protection of anonymity necessary for
discussing personal problems; it offers both closeness and
neutrality. The opportunity to speak freely, knowing that
someone is listening, someone who has time and yet doesn't
press for a decision, increases relaxation during a massage. This
in turn reduces inner tension and cramping. A massage often has
the effect of promoting both external relief and inner release.
Familiarity with the specific circumstances can make rehabilitation easier for both the patient and the therapist.

# Back Muscles as a Final Link in a Stress Chain

For the symptom of back pain, there are so many different
contexts of questions and so many oblique factors such as diet,
life-style, and emotional influences that a comprehensive view
and evaluation is difficult indeed. The origin of each person's
back complaints is based on the condition of his back and on a
unique group of contributing factors. Therefore the emphasis on
specific complaints and causes ultimately leading to pain are
different in each person. Faulty posture may not in itself be the
pain-causing factor but, combined with an emotional factor, it

*When has
the critical
point been
exceeded?*

can be a last link in a chain of risk factors that exceeds the limits
of the bearable for the back muscles. The trouble might have
been initiated by the stress of a car ride, getting chilled, or lifting
a heavy object that exceeded the critical limits.

For these reasons, each diagnosis applies to one specific back.
Diagnosis is a kind of symbiosis since each person has to put up
with his own back that participates in all he does. How a person
walks, sits, sleeps, what he feels and experiences—be it anger,
happiness, anxiety, fear or aggression—all react on that extraordinarily sensitive individual organ, the back.

15

# The Back—Stepchild of Preventive Medicine

Many laypersons may know a little something about discs, but almost nothing about back muscles. Even though it is muscular pain rather than nerve pain or pain caused by physical changes in the joints that plagues us most often, only slight consideration is given to muscles. Preventive medicine represents one of the most significant advances of modern therapy in general and is one of the reasons for longevity. A sensible life-style and regular examinations, or preventive medicine, are of increasing importance.

*A test for muscle fitness*

But notice what a preventive examination includes: first, the heart and circulatory system; then the liver and kidney functions, and tests for blood sugar content. A check for cancer cells is also made. All of this is routine, but as Professor Hans Kraus, one of the pioneers in orthopedic preventive medicine who created the "Muscle Fitness Test," justly complains, an examination of the back and the status of the musculature is seldom part of the checkup. Almost without exception, the back is only examined when it causes pain.

# Posture—Mirror of the Emotional and Physical State

What are back pains actually? Almost every person has experienced them. There is hardly anyone who at some time has not experienced pain in the small of the back, neck, or between the shoulder blades, or has not had a pain radiating into the shoulders, leg or head, or whose back has not hurt from bending. Sometimes upon getting up in the morning a person may feel as if his back has a hangover. Evidently the back is much more sensitive than its robust muscle structure would indicate, and it reacts to everything that affects the whole organism. Seemingly nothing gets by it unnoticed. Often people are wrongly admonished to "stand stiffly" and to "use backbone" in dealing with particularly difficult situations. The

*Reflection of attitude*

reminder, though, "to straighten up" is not merely an empty old saying. All such formulations express in various forms the idea

16

that there is a connection between the back and psychic reactions. The back in effect is a mirror of the physical and emotional state, the inner and external attitude of a person.


# The Back as a Functional Unity

What is the back, what does it look like and what does it include? The question appears simple but is far more encompassing than it seems. If a person sits on a stool, tilts his head forward, and puts his arms in his lap, the position expresses both in appearance and in function his back's attitude. This is important to know since this whole area, even though made up of many different components (the rear wall of the pelvis, the spinal column, the rear section of the ribs, the neck and shoulders) reacts as a working unit. We therefore speak of the functional unity of the back. Most movement impulses are initiated here, and every change or disturbance in the peripheral area is expressed here. Any imbalance or deviation from the norm produces an echo effect on the back. Why, though, does such a compact organ as the back react so sensitively to demands from the environment and why does it wear out so quickly? Why is it that leg muscles do not feel their age, while back muscles do? Why is a forty-year-old knuckle or ankle joint not worn out or painful, while a vertebral joint often is at thirty? Why is a disc more sensitive than a meniscus?

*The back is a sensitive organ*

From this perspective, we will try to give a diagnostic explanation to all those who suffer from the symptom of back pain and some advice to those who are not yet or are no longer patients. Doctors usually have too little time to explain this sub-acute medical area to the insufficiently informed layman.

a joint undergoing only the beginning of change that may a.d.

# 2. The Significance of Pain

## Pain Intensity—Pain Quality

To understand the causes of back pain, it is first necessary to know what pain actually is, how it feels, what causes it, and which connective tissue is capable of registering it.

*Pain cannot be measured*

Pain cannot be scientifically and precisely measured. Nor can its intensity be measured. There is not even an immediate relationship between the magnitude of a pain-causing injury (noxa) and the intensity of the pain, and as a consequence pain can only be described subjectively. Pain, however, is always comprised of two components—the pain-causing stimulus as the transmitter of pain, and the feeling, or the consciousness, of the person affected.

*The phe-nomenon of imagining pain*

A severely worn, almost stiff joint may initially produce relatively little pain in comparison with a very sensitive spot on a joint undergoing only the beginning of change that may not show up on x-ray. But if a patient sees an x-ray of his knee joint that has undergone radical change as a result of arthritis, his pain might increase significantly because he is now able to visualize his ailment. Conversely, the pain might lessen if the change he observed on the x-ray were minor.

Back pain does not always correspond to objective clinical findings. For example, a tight, tense-as-a-board back might be quiet for a long time, whereas a single cramped muscle fiber can produce an unbearable pulling pain on a bone's periosteum which is highly sensitive.*

---

*Periosteum is a membrane of fibrous tissue containing many blood vessels and sensitive fibers that covers all bones.

Even though pain intensity is only measurable subjectively, the quality of pain can be described as mute, piercing, light, or cutting. A pain felt on the outer skin, for example, is generally light, sharp, or cutting; such superficial pain can be localized and usually abates in a relatively brief time.

Pain arising from a deeper source such as from the bones, muscles, and connective tissue is dull, gnawing, and difficult to localize because it radiates into the surrounding area. This kind of pain does not abate and there is no getting used to it (adaptation is missing). This characteristic distinguishes deep pain from superficial pain. Deep pain can be manifested in an area totally different from its origin—somewhere on the surface of the body, for example. It can project itself onto a different part of the body. A slipped disc can therefore cause pain in the leg, and a headache or a pain in the arm may have its origin in the cervical vertebral column.

Pain caused by deep-seated organs such as intestines or glands, is similar to deep pain in its quality. It radiates, and the sufferer does not become habituated to it. Through a nervous coupling effect that does not pass through the brain but only through the spinal column, the pain from an organ can affect a certain area of skin belonging to the particular organ, causing it to be oversensitive. These nervous-reflex skin areas of the affected organs are named after their discoverer and are termed Head's Zones. They are mainly important because the organ-skin coupling can be reversed, and the deep-seated organ can be reached therapeutically through the affected skin area.

# Individual Pain Tolerance

Pain sensitivity, or the pain threshold, varies in each individual. Moreover, the ability to tolerate pain varies from person to person and also depends on the momentary emotional condition of the person when pain strikes. The person may be utterly at the mercy of pain if his general condition is poor and his psychological state unstable. On the other hand, pain may be easy to tolerate and to ignore if the person is in good condition and in a good frame of mind. An injured football player, for example, who confidently dashed to the goal line will hardly be aware of any pain, whereas his opponent may writhe in pain on the field. It also must be taken into consideration that pain often acquires an aggressive thrust and heightened intensity among children—and in certain situations among adults also—as a result of a particular goal or purpose to be achieved by it.

# Pain as the Body's Warning Signal

*Pain as a lifesaving alarm signal*

Pain is the warning signal of the body, an indication of a disturbance or an injury. A noted physiologist, H. Rein, stated concerning the usefulness of pain and its place in everyone's life, "Pain ultimately protects man from constant harm and is indispensable for normal life."

# Pain Affects the Total Organism

If pain is felt on the skin's surface, we react automatically by withdrawing the hand or foot with a jerking motion or by turning the head, depending on the type and location of the pain. The rapidity with which this protective or defensive reaction takes place is only possible because of learned processes that occur automatically (reflexes). These processes are transmitted from the point of injury through the spinal column to the brain stem and from there to the cerebral cortex, where it is recognized and immediately switched to the motor defense mechanism. This area of the brain stem influences and controls all vital processes. It links and, as needed, synchronizes the vegetative (autonomic) nervous system, the circulatory center, the breathing center and other vital regulatory processes.

When a pain stimulus occurs, the area of the brain stem functions as a reloading point that both transmits the warning to the consciousness and activates the autonomic nervous system. The autonomic nervous system in turn reacts by causing faster breathing, a quickened heart rate, and perspiration. In this manner, the whole body reacts to pain. Hence sciatica is more than a pain; it can be connected with a real feeling of illness. A migraine is not only a headache, it also involves a drop in blood pressure, greater sensitivity of the eyes to light, and an intense feeling of nausea that can lead to vomiting. Finding the cause of such deep pain is often difficult. Anyone who has had pain in the small of the back, neck, or shoulders, knows how long it takes to trace the cause and to alleviate the attack.

# Pain Sensitivity of Connective Tissue

Not all organs and connective tissues of the body are equally sensitive to pain, so the important questions in trying to understand the phenomenon of back pain are: Which constituent part of the back can feel pain? Which connective tissue can feel pain? How and through what does back pain come about?

Evidently the skin covering the body cavities such as the pleura, the peritoneum, and the meninges are very susceptible to pain. This is also true of thè membrane covering the bones, the periosteum. In contrast, the bone itself, especially the bone cortex—and for some curious reason the brain—have no sensitivity to pain at all.

# Can Muscles Feel Pain?

Muscle fibers are insensitive to pain, but under certain circumstances they can become sensitive to pain. Their pain sensitivity depends on their metabolism, particularly on an adequate supply of oxygen. The pain threshold of muscles is exceeded when there is a disproportion of oxygen supply and demand and poor elimination of metabolic waste. This seems to be the case in a prolonged cramping of the musculature. A continual state of heightened tension in the back muscles, for

*Hypersensitivity of the back muscles to pain*

example, impairs the metabolism of these muscles to such an extent that the pain threshold is exceeded. It can even produce a hypersensitivity to pain in these muscles, which then causes the whole back to hurt.

Such long-term heightening of the basic tension in entire groups of muscles may have come into being as a defensive tensing against deep organ pain—as, for example, during an acute attack of appendicitis, or during great physical exertion, particularly in connection with cold temperatures and in situations of emotional stress. Intellectual activity or emotional

22

turmoil increases the metabolism not only in the brain but in the entire organism as a result of heightened tension of the musculature.*

# Muscle Strain As a Result of Emotional Stress

*Improving muscle tone*

Two English researchers, Sainsbury and Gibson, using electric action current measurements, tested various persons who had muscle strain caused by emotional stress. The results showed that during an emotionally strenuous conversation the muscle tone of the subjects became measurably heightened. This tension diminished rapidly among subjects whose muscles were rested, elastic, and physiologically sound. They could spontaneously loosen their muscles, and their muscles regenerated quickly. But for those whose muscles were cramped prior to the experiment, the conversation caused further cramping which became even worse after the experiment was completed. They were in a stress situation, they were no longer able to relax, and the ability of the muscles to recover vanished.

Evidently it is primarily the metabolism in cramped muscles that is disturbed, resulting in a lowered pain threshold. This basic knowledge concerning the effect of metabolism and oxygen supply on muscle pain is indispensable in determining treatment and in inducing relaxation of a cramped back musculature.

# Muscle Pain Due to Lack of Oxygen

A muscle requires an abundant supply of oxygen in order to be efficient, elastic, and free of pain. Where does it get its oxygen supply? The muscles themselves have their own store of oxygen, but the supply is small, adequate only for a 100-meter dash. In order to function for a longer period of time, breathing and circulation must supply the increase. The breathing becomes

---

*Muscle tone is the amount of tension in a muscle.

23

deeper and the heart must supply more blood, otherwise, the muscles will tire quickly and react with heightened tension and cramping and above all with pain. This explains the muscle pain in Buerger's disease (leg muscles do not receive sufficient blood flow due to thickening arterial walls.) It also explains the cramps in the calves of a long-distance runner (his breathing at the end of a run is no longer able to meet his great need of oxygen).

*Leg muscle pain resulting from Buerger's disease*

# Restricted Blood Flow Due to Muscle Cramping

It is unnecessary to go so far afield or to seek special cases to illustrate the relationship between oxygen supply and muscular metabolism and the resulting pain sensitivity of the musculature. A back muscle that is stiff as a ramrod, often involving a whole muscle group, undergoes greater metabolic change and has a greater need for oxygen than a normal back muscle. After all, the muscle is physiologically at work. But the arterial blood supply to such a muscle—i.e., its provision of fresh, oxygen-rich blood—is especially poor. The cramped back muscle, because of its great tension, cuts itself off from the blood needed for supply, recuperation, and removal of metabolic waste. The muscle clamps off the small capillaries and thus strangles its own metabolic exchange of substances. The breathing movement of the chest cavity, which is the condition for a supply of oxygen, is tightened; when this happens, a virtual muscle corset is created. Under these conditions, it is easy to see that only a little extra something is needed—cold, physical exertion, a wrong move, or emotional stress—to cause pain in such tensed, cramped muscles.

*Removal of metabolic waste*

# Sore Muscles

Sore muscles are less the result of inadequate metabolism, as was long assumed, than of extensive mechanical overexertion. The ability of an untrained muscle to contract varies, and not all are equally able to contract. As a result, those muscle fibers particularly capable of contraction can compel the weaker fibers

*Possible causes*

24

to cooperate to the point of breaking them. The resulting pain or sore muscle is therefore caused by numerous fine tears within the individual muscle fibers.

# Periosteum Pain Due to a Pulled Muscle

*Tennis elbow*

Periosteum pain is not actually a muscle pain. The pain is released by muscles as a result of a persistent pull by a cramped muscle strand on the periosteum of a bone of the locomotor system. The point attacked by such an irritation is the transition of the muscle tendon into the periosteum. Here the tendon blends with the periosteum, and the fibers mesh and blend into bony tissue. The pain of tennis elbow, for example, is the result of such a pull, often caused by overuse of musculature or by untrained musculature. This is also the origin of much shoulder-arm stiffness *(page 61)* or a hip-joint arthropathy *(page 58)*. Even the pain sensitivity of many spinal processes in the spinal column results from constant muscular pull.

# 3. Back Pains and Their Causes

## Symptoms and Syndromes

A symptom is a characteristic feature of the course of a particular disease. Disease can be recognized and diagnosed from a number of typical symptoms. Atypical symptoms of a clinical picture can also, however, make diagnosis difficult, especially since one and the same symptom can be manifested in different diseases. Pain in the small of the back, for example, is a symptom for a variety of clinical pictures, or syndromes. It can be the result of a severe gynecological problem, a crushed disc, severe constipation, or of a kidney disorder. Severe headaches can be caused by migraines, eye trouble, too low or too high blood pressure, or a brain tumor.

*Pain in the small of the back is a symptom*

A syndrome is a combination of symptoms that originally belong together and are manifested in one and the same disturbance for which they are typical. Various indications of different organs and tissues are thus involved. Taken all together, these indications yield a clinical picture, or what is called a syndrome. The medical profession occasionally also uses the term, complex of symptoms.

## Diagnosis: Myogelosis

Myogelosis, or hardening of the muscles, is a symptom. The

condition is a characteristic sign of strained or overworked back musculature. The causes are extremely varied and can occur in numerous syndromes. These knotty thickenings are found in the back musculature of almost every adult, but they may not always cause problems, especially in the beginning. They are, however, a sign that a muscle's metabolism is no longer functioning properly. If the condition worsens, the basic tension of the muscle fibers is heightened and the hardened muscles are felt to be painful knots.

*Tangible muscle hardening*

Myogelosis is found particularly often in those muscle groups whose strong fibers run diagonally from the inner edge of the shoulder blades to the spinal column. Myogelosis is also often present in the thick neck muscle whose fibers spread out in various directions from the back of the head across the throat, neck and shoulders, dispatching a bundle of muscle fibers to each spinal process of vertebrae in the area of the thorax. These muscle hardenings can literally be grasped in the process of massage, often prompting the patient to ask with some astonishment whether it is cartilage. Such a tightly pulled muscle strand with embedded myogelosis often jumps back and forth like a taut string across the bony edge of the shoulder blade and then can not only be touched but heard as well. These hardenings in the muscles are, like many degenerative changes of the back, manifestations of aging that have no necessary relationship to chronological age. The term *degenerative* primarily signifies a development of an organ or organ tissue that deviates from the physiological norm and deteriorates in a particular manner. The course followed by such irregular development is typical. Its consistent intervening stages and recurrent signals make it recognizable.

Such degeneration, especially of those muscle fibers that have poor blood supply, causes a loosening of tissue and a partial dissolution of the muscle substance in the muscle cells. The contractile substance characteristic of muscle elasticity becomes clumpy. In such dissolution, connective tissue fibers mix in with metabolic waste and thereby cause increasing thickening, or myogelosis. The small capillaries that supply blood to the single muscle fibers cannot prevent this advancing process. They are also affected, their walls thicken, become impassable and waste away. Thus the metabolic state of these muscles steadily worsens, the muscle loses elasticity and becomes taut. Myogelosis becomes painful when the total metabolic state of

28

the host muscle deteriorates to the extent that it lacks oxygen. A vicious cycle is thus set up. Overexertion of a muscle caused by physical overexertion, emotional stress, a tendency toward weak tissues, or a combination of all these factors heighten tension in the musculature, which then slows down metabolism. This leads to structural changes of the muscle fibers, the formation of muscle hardenings, and deterioration of capillaries in the area. This results in poor blood supply, a further cramping of the musculature, and an increase, enlargement, and hardening of the myogelosis. The pain threshold of the affected muscle is quickly exceeded. Then the body, in a last-ditch attempt to avoid pain, adds a defensive tensing of the muscle. It attempts to rest the muscle through cramping.

*Vicious cycle*       Relief necessitates breaking the vicious cycle. The goal must be to elasticize the affected muscles again, to reduce their tension, and to stimulate their metabolism—in short, to provide them with the much-needed oxygen for all these processes.

# Diagnosis: Rheumatism of the Soft Tissues

*Syndrome*       Rheumatism of the soft tissues is not a clearly defined
*not clearly*       syndrome. The term is used for all painful muscle processes in
*defined*       which the origin of the pain is unknown. It refers to complaints which sometimes are manifested as painful centers, at other times as radiating pain which darts about mostly in the back or neck musculature and which lacks specific characteristics. Although inflammatory processes are often mentioned, rheumatism of the soft tissues—with the exception of pain— lacks the classic symptoms of swelling, reddening, and warmth. These manifestations are therefore often called degenerative inflammatory processes. But this term is not completely accurate either, since it does not reflect changes in the blood count, the presence of a rheumatoid factor in the blood, or an acceleration of blood sedimentation—i.e., the typical symptoms of a genuine rheumatic disease. These descriptions simply apply to a disease process in those disturbed muscle areas containing myogelosis that are tense and, most significantly, painful.

29

# Diagnosis: Muscular Bracing of the Back

## Why so many people suffer from spasms

Cramping evidently always results from a disproportion between load and load capacity—regardless of whether the disproportion is physical, mental, or emotional. Since the load capacity is different in each individual, it is impossible to establish a norm. Some emotionally robust persons are physically frail and conversely some physically robust persons are emotionally frail.

*Sleep dis-*
*turbances as*
*a result*
Then, too, the pressure to achieve experienced by everyone in our society includes job demands, social life, the environment, the fight against aging, and the compulsion to remain young, maintain healthy potency, creativity, and dynamism. A great deal is expected from each of us, and we react differently to the expectations imposed on us. Two common symptoms of this overexertion are inability to sleep and back pain. Inability to sleep is only mentioned here because of the heightened muscle tone that results from the nerve-racking experience of insomnia.

Next to heart and circulatory disease, cramping of the back musculature and its related complaints is the most common ailment of our era. If the definition of health from the World Health Organization (WHO) is applied, "a condition of complete physical, mental, emotional, and social well-being not attained merely by the absence of disease and weakness," then it must be assumed that very few people are truly healthy.

## Does school make children ill?

*School*
*children with*
*back*
*problems*
Back complaints know no age limit. Back pains among students in their final year of high school or even children of age ten and twelve are no longer a rarity in a physiotherapist's office. Formerly the most important consideration in diagnosing young patients was based on the assumption that postural weakness leads to poor posture and postural injury. Today, pure muscle cramping independent of orthopedic causes is as frequent.

If the statement, "school makes children ill," is true, then the major reason is poor posture. We will return to this topic later *(page 53)*. The pressure to achieve that is exerted on children

30

stems primarily from society rather than from school. The demands made on young people to achieve social status, success, a quick promotion, to acquire objects that will lend them prestige, and a strong overrating of academic learning are all social values indiscriminately transmitted by parents and children. Children are scolded and admonished to stand up straight as a sign of achievement but their weak, untrained backs cannot stand the strain. Exams as such do not cause back aches, but the fact that they must be passed with a certain grade, that future social success is made to depend on them, is the decisive factor that causes muscle tone even among children to exceed the pain threshold.

## Speed is a stress factor

The situation is no different at the work place. Today a frighteningly large number of workers retire early because of disorders related to back problems. It is also now clear that physical stress has been overestimated as a cause of work-related back problems. It is also clear that there has been an overreliance on a strictly orthopedic approach. Increased mechanization brought with it the hope that back muscles would be greatly relieved of stress. This has not happened, however, It is now known that mental concentration—waiting for the right moment to press a button, the task of carefully monitoring instruments, keeping up with the tempo of a machine—demands more of muscles than many activities merely involving physical labor.

*Mechaniza-*
*tion is a*
*dead-end*
*street*

## Concentration instead of body movement

*Driving can*
*cause*
*cramps*

The stress exerted on our backs from driving a car does not primarily come from poor posture (this is of importance to the discs, as we will see later). The vibrations and jolts received while driving would also not be so detrimental were it not for the strain on the back muscles as a result of the intense concentration necessary for driving at high speed. Speed also places too great a strain on our sensory organs. Many attempts have been made to test and examine the relationship between speed and blood pressure, between tempo and pulse beat, between exhaust fumes and breathing. The back muscles most

31

clearly reveal the effect of speed and concentration on the whole organism.

A case history: a strong, young, muscular woman in apparent good health with all the prerequisites for a healthy back musculature. She lived in the country, had healthy growing children, and a good marriage. She came to me for physiotherapy treatments. She complained of very taut neck and shoulder muscles accompanied by severe pain that radiated into the arm and almost impeded every movement. She responded quickly to treatment, especially to massage of the fibrous tissues, and her circulation improved markedly. The complaints abated. But she soon suffered a relapse, which we both agreed to be the result of her washing windows. With the next severe attack, however, I found the real reason for the relapse: she was racing her car over a 300-mile distance at an average speed of 100mph in order to save thirty minutes. All her relapses during the course of my treatment were the result of excessive driving speeds.

*Street traffic and aggression*

Laws to curtail speed rarely have as their motive the health impact of speed. But the stress that speeders create for others by ignoring signs and lights, tailgating, and aggressive behavior should be considered. People unaccustomed to such hectic circumstances become overexerted. They react with back pain, dizziness, or even heart attacks.

**Occupational stress**

Muscular bracing of the back among many working women is less the result of physical overexertion than a reaction to the multiplicity of their tasks, the fragmentation of concentration between job, home, husband, children, and school. People usually can more readily cope with strenuous work than the coordination of three or four jobs in a given period of time. We also may tend to overlook the telephone as a stress factor in an office. Although an experienced secretary no longer jumps in response to the aggressive sound of the ring, her autonomic nervous system reacts each time without her being aware of it. A telephone mercilessly interrupts every task, every thought, every mood, and always demands a small new beginning, a piecing-together of the thread of concentration interrupted by the sound of the bell. A still worse stress situation exists in a

*Robot*
*atmosphere*
*of large*
*offices*

large office where many typists use headsets to work on topics incomprehensible to them that were dictated by invisible voices. They have no possibility of communication, agreement, or even of hearing the expression of thanks. In this situation the inhumanity of a robot society is scarcely a step away, and backaches are the ineluctable consequence.

Stress factors are also present in the higher echelons of large companies. Here, however, they merely assume a different appearance. Their origin is rivalry, professional jealousy, the fear of not being able to keep pace with technical innovations, the fear of aging, and the constant battle of maintaining a feeling of self-esteem.

The need to adjust to an alien tempo, whether of machines, assembly lines, dictaphones, a conference timetable, or the greater work ability of a younger colleague, tightens back muscles and demands more of them than a car seat that is too soft, an uncomfortable desk chair, or physical labor.

*Emotional*
*reactions*
*can cause*
*cramps*

We have said earlier that strong emotional reactions can tense the back. It is especially difficult to come to grips with the cause of such tensing since it is necessary to live with the people and situations that give rise to the problem. Family members, a spouse, co-workers, and close neighbors are often involved. The tension can be triggered by cramped living quarters, noise, or too much heat at the place of work, by depression, aggression, or by financial worries. In all these instances, physiotherapy in combination with medical treatment can bring relief. Even the possibility of a discussion, perhaps during treatment, and the knowledge that someone else is aware of these stresses can be helpful.

What is it, though, in the body that produces these tensions? Which mechanisms transmit the feeling to the affected organ—in this instance to the muscle?

### The transmission mechanism of mind-muscle

*Influence of*
*autonomic*
*nervous*
*system*

The influence exerted by the brain stem on all life processes, including the autonomic nervous system, has already been discussed. The brain stem can be conceived as a switching and distribution point that establishes the connection between consciousness (i.e., the cerebrum and its cortex, which is primarily the locus of our intellectual capabilities) and our emotional attitude. One of the functions of the vegetative nervous system is to control the degree of intensity of our responses. It always has the possibility of stimulating or of dampening our responses, depending upon which part of its components gains the upper hand. The parasympathetic components restrain life processes, while the sympathetic components trigger and speed up the processes.

The autonomic nervous system also serves to regulate the hormone-producing glands. What is important in this context is primarily the suprarenal gland, along with its adrenal medulla and adrenal cortex, and also the pituitary. Their prime function is to supply adrenalin to the circulatory system. Like the sympathetic nervous system, adrenalin has a stimulating effect.

*Basic tension of the skeletal musculature*

The interplay of these systems influences breathing, pulse rate, and blood pressure. It also serves to regulate muscle tone, the basic tension of the skeletal musculature. For this reason, every upsetting emotional event triggers some fireworks, and this in turn can set in motion a series of chain reactions. In each instance, it is the autonomic nervous system that supplies the impulse, this is then followed by the activation of the sympathetic nervous system, which causes the suprarenal and pituitary to release a greater supply of adrenalin into the blood stream. The blood pressure rises, the pulse rate increases, and breathing is forced. Perspiration flows, the muscles become tense, and their tone is heightened. All these phases can be observed by watching a cat as it eyes a dog from a safe distance. The process of activation can be observed from the moment the cat first notices the dog to the climax, when all its muscles are tensed for the leap to flee or to attack. We, too, daily experience several comparable periods of agitation, which usually end, however, without either flight or attack. Our emotional hide, so to speak, usually smoothes out again, since our typical reaction is one of adaptation and our typical escape is repression. The heightened muscle tone remains, however, as the expression of an inner readiness for alarm.

## Syndrome of overstrain

The reaction described above is similar to that experienced by the organism during physical exertion. Here also there is increased breathing, quickened pulse rate, an increase in blood

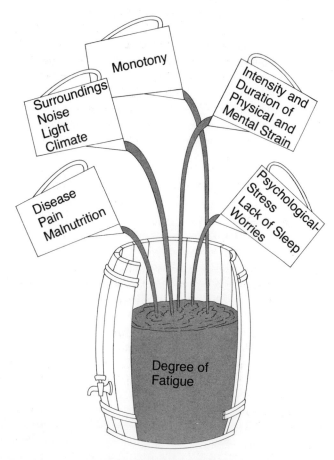

*"Barrel of Fatigue."* If the barrel overflows, the result is general exhaustion or overexertion syndrome.

*The muscula-
ture as the
central organ
to react*

pressure and muscle tension. If physical labor must be done under emotional pressure—with a quarrelsome co-worker or an unpleasant superior, under time pressure, or during sports competition when the pressure of too great expectations can cause psychic stress—the results in terms of heightened physical and emotional stress can easily be measured. Our body, like a concave radar disc, collects all our responses to these burdens and transmits them to the central reactive organ, the muscula-ture. The metabolism must deal with every burden, regardless of the source.

35

## Metabolism responds to stress

Proof that the organism does indeed react strongly to stress can be shown by the increased manifestation of specific metabolic products in the blood and urine. These products—as, for example, lactic acids—originate in part from endogenous oxidation processes. Or they are hormonal waste products, such as vanillin-mandelic acids from suprarenal adrenalin. Evidence of these substances is one possibility of really measuring emotional work and of identifying it as a burden. Mainly, though, these tests reveal that the body is strained by events in which it is involved only passively and emotionally, and these tests also demonstrate that emotional work is strenuous. In this respect, the body's response is comparable to a spectator's response at an exciting football game or a movie thriller, or to a passenger's experience while riding in a speeding car. For these reasons, it is advisable after an exhausting event to relax physically until the autonomic nervous system has returned to normal. A walk in the fresh air or a short bicycle ride will serve to let off steam and avoid going to bed when one's metabolism is functioning at high capacity.

*Overexertion due to emotional strain*

Little fantasy is required to imagine the frame of mind of many children as they are being sent to bed at night. When already tired, they are permitted to watch a movie on T.V., which they experience emotionally more strongly than an adult would. In addition, their efforts to concentrate on what is for them overtaxing intellectual content make them still more tense. At this point, there is no opportunity for them to work off either the emotional or the physical overexertion. Many parents nonetheless wonder why their children lie awake for hours, even though they were put to bed at an early hour.

*TV and tension*

## Purely physical overstrain

There is, naturally, purely physical overexertion resulting from physical labor or exertion. Many jobs require hard physical labor, and some young people are not physically ready for the work they do. Long hours spent sitting still in school and doing homework are also a great ordeal for the vertebrae and back musculature.

The damage caused by physical overstrain is primarily

reflected in the fibrous and supporting tissue—i.e., in ligaments, bones, and joints. If there is a disproportion between their strength and the demand made on them, they wear out early. We will discuss changes in the spinal column and in discs in greater detail in a later passage.

In this connection, let me briefly describe an incident. The use of anabolics by female athletes is not without danger. Anabolics have an effect analogous to male sex hormones and are used to promote muscle growth. These hormones promote the development of masculine proportions of muscle that are too strong for the more slight female skeletal system. Because of the pull then exerted on the muscle, ligaments and tendons can be torn and the bone itself can be damaged. Due to accumulated physical and emotional strain, this condition can persist and develop into an independent syndrome often encountered in physiotherapeutic treatment.

# Diagnosis: Vegetative Dystonia

Vegetative dystonia belongs in our discussion, since it also involves an overexertion syndrome. But it has a much wider scope than the syndrome of back pain and primarily involves vegetative false regulations of the heart and circulatory process.

A similar reaction is at the root of all overexertion syndromes. The body mobilizes its emergency reserves and tries to overcompensate for the drain on its strength in order to meet all the other demands made on it. An overexerted organism can thus live on credit for a time, but then it collapses without warning. The body's response resembles that of an athlete who uses medication that makes it possible for him to surpass his normal strength. When his reserves are used up, he collapses.

This condition is usually less dramatic than the example cited, because it exists in varying degrees and in constantly changing combinations of symptoms. At times the more nervous, mechanical signs of circulatory irregularities prevail such as palpitations, extra-systolic beats, a stumbling of the heart rhythm; at other times, muscular cramping prevails. But all the danger signals are present although they are present in various degrees of intensity.

A typical example of the piling up of physical and emotional stress factors that result in vegetative dystonia—heart and circulatory instability, sleep disturbances and muscle cramping—can be illustrated in the case of a patient I recently treated.

*A metal worker*

A metal worker had done hard physical labor all his life. He had spent 8 hours a day standing, bending, and lifting objects. He suffered a dislocated disc (prolapse) with a severe sciatic syndrome when he was 50. Even though his strong musculature could take a lot, his back was severely overstrained. Because of increasing neurological complaints—tickling and numbness of the foot and a motoric weakness of the leg musculature—he was finally operated on after two months of conservative treatment in various clinics, and the disc that was pressing on the sciatic nerve was removed. The operation went well, the patient recovered quickly, and my treatment began after his release from the hospital (about four weeks after surgery). After another four weeks, he was completely free of pain and only registered a slight numbness in his foot. The time to return to work approached, prompting typical worries and questions: how will his back and discs respond to the unaccustomed stress or work? Is he going to be able to do any lifting, bending, or standing for long periods? Will he be able physically to put in an 8-hour day? His job does not permit him to get used to working slowly; it requires him to be fit from the first day, able to maintain the tempo, carry his expected work load, and to keep up. He must, therefore, adapt himself to the rhythm of a healthy person. Although actually healthy, he is out of training after having been away from work for four months. A week's vacation still due him permitted a short delay in returning to work. Three days before time to resume work, he developed difficulty in sleeping,

*Anxiety is registered in the neck*

suffered a loss of appetite, had attacks of tachycardia, and moved about restlessly during the night. In addition, severe backaches developed before he returned to work. These were not in the area treated by surgery but were instead in the area between the shoulder blades where psychological tension is usually felt. The emotional stress, the feeling of inadequacy, the fear of not being able to keep up with the pace of work, the fear of losing the job, of no longer being able at age 50 to be competitive was so severe that he was affected precisely as if he had done hard physical labor. He was vegetatively exhausted.

38

**Convalescence problems**

*From zero to full capacity*

In such cases, a slow increase in activity should be made possible. A chance for adjustment, perhaps by working only half a day should be arranged. The necessity of going from zero to full capacity, of having to adjust to the working tempo of a healthy individual by having to stand or sit at a desk or cash register for 8 hours creates immense emotional stress.

# Diagnosis: LVC-Syndrome

LVC stands for lumbar vertebral column syndrome. It occurs when there is an injury or a functional distrubance in the area of the lumbar vertebrae. The syndrome includes many symptoms that can be found in various combinations and in different degrees of severity.

*Boring pain as a symptom*

The cause of complaints in most cases is a worn-out, used-up disc that causes a deep boring pain in the small of the back. Such pain should be a signal that it is time to consult a physician.

All disc deterioration syndromes typically occur regardless of age. They are only noticed when they cause pain; they have a tendency to heal themselves. This topic will be discussed later in some detail.

Although there are other reasons for pain in this area, disc problems will be discussed first because of their importance and frequency. It is necessary to know the function of a disc, because only then is it possible to understand how and why it wears out. So much has been written and said about discs that to state that it connects two vertebrae is almost superfluous.

**Wear and tear in the area of the lumbar vertebrae**

Manifestations of wear and tear in the area of the lumbar vertebrae are naturally very frequent, because this section of the spinal column is particularly mobile. It is also subjected to balancing out substantial weights and must endure the greatest burden of pressure. There is a distinct curve at the point of transition in the lumbar vertebral column to the sacrum, and it is

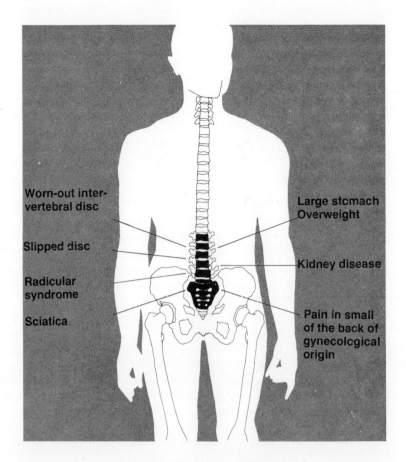

*Lumbar spinal column and sacrum.* Area affected by LVC syndrome. It is here that disc problems most frequently occur. The illustrations shows which complaints originate here and which factors are involved in this occurrence.

here that most disc incidents occur. This curve is located at a functionally critical point; since the lumbar vertebrae are very flexible while the sacral vertebrae and sacrum are utterly rigid, they are grown together to form a block—i.e., to form the bony, compact sacrum. Ninety-five percent of all disc problems originate at this particularly menaced spot, which is between the 4th and 5th lumbar vertebrae (L4 and L5) and the 5th lumbar (L5) and 1st sacral vertebrae (S1) (Brunngraber).

Frequency and localization of disc problems:
between L1 and L2—0.2%
between L2 and L3—1.4%
between L3 and L4—2.9%
between L4 and L5—48%
between L5 and S1—47.2%
between S1 and S2—0.4%

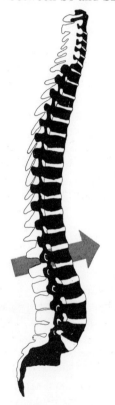

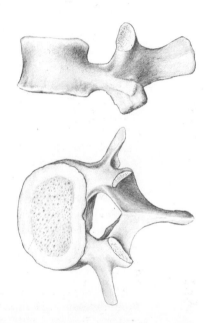

*Side view of the entire spinal column. Above right:* side view of single lumbar vertebral bodies. *Lower right:* cross section of lumbar vertebral bodies.

**Aging is not an illness for discs**

The term, manifestation of wear and tear, is often overused in connection with discs. It is easily equated with diseased and painful conditions and is used for every normal biological aging process. Perhaps the term, signs of aging, should preferably be used, since in the majority of cases what is involved are physiological changes or the aging of tissues which are registered in the entire organism.

*Aging does
not mean
being sick*

Aging does not necessarily imply illness.

It is also always necessary to be aware that the visible degree of wear and tear does not correspond to the resulting intensity of complaints. Complaints arising from such tissue changes can be lessened or alleviated completely, without any change being reflected in the x-ray that visibly shows detrition of the bone.

**Self-healing is possible**

*Forced
retirement*

Many backaches, especially in the area of the small of the back, disappear in old age by themselves. A certain stiffness of this area results in involuntary immobility, thereby causing acute irritation to diminish. Or the complaints may diminish if the excrescences of intervertebral disc tissue are located where there is sufficient room to avoid pressing on a nerve. A patient who comes to a doctor or therapist, stating "I have had a disc problem for years," will still have a disc problem even if he leaves free of complaint after 10 or 15 treatments. But he can live with the disc. The muscle cramping has abated, he is able to breathe deeply again, his muscles get more oxygen, they are free of pain.

**Tissues and loss of fluids**

General signs of aging of the organs and tissues include a loss of fluid, evidently resulting from a change in ability to absorb water, particularly by fibrous tissue and its specific proteins. If the smooth skin of an infant is compared with the wrinkled, flabby skin of a seventy-year old, the extent of the general loss of fluid is apparent. All other tissues of the organism also undergo many changes with aging. To summarize, it is possible to speak of a general loss of elasticity, particularly in the fibrous and supporting tissue, of calcification process in some tendons and of decalcification in much-used bones. That is why, for instance, old people are more prone to a fractured hip than young people.

This physiological aging process can occur more rapidly from a number of factors: great strain, a disproportion in the rudimentary quality of the tissue and the strength required of the tissue, an unhealthy way of life, lack of training, one-sided strain in an asymmetric body condition, or from overweight.

42

## The problem of disc metabolism

*Problems in obtaining nourishment*

Although discs have an important function and are subject to strenuous demands, they are among the most poorly nourished tissues of the body. Their upright position at the outset makes providing them with nutritive substance difficult. During the embryonic state and during the first few years of life, they are well fed by their own blood supply. These wither away to nothing by age four. Thereafter the discs are fed only through diffusion (Loeweneck). This means that the metabolic exchange takes place through the cell walls while the fluid moves from the stronger to the weaker concentration. If the concentration of metabolic waste is too high, it is emptied into the surrounding fluid; if the concentration of nourishment in the surrounding area is greater than that of the disc tissue, it can penetrate the tissue and hence diffuse.

*Pull and pressure demand*

These processes are additionally supported by the burdening and unburdening of the discs through the stress of pull or pressure. Every movement, every change of position, every weight gain affects disc metabolism. For example, the intake of substance while in a relaxed, supine position almost approximates a suction effect, while intake from a standing position almost presses the fluid out of the discs (Krämer). That is why it is important for the discs to have a fequent change of position and stress and why movement of the spinal column is important if the discs are to receive their supply of nourishment. It also explains why sitting and standing are such a burden on the discs, for in these positions they cannot be nourished.

## The special strain of sitting

It has been established that the strain on the discs is much greater while sitting than standing. When standing, the natural curvature of the spine distributes pressure. For this reason, sitting still in school is a torture for children and for their discs; therefore desks designed to be used while standing would be physiologically preferable. Our discs also suffer when we phone a co-worker next door or one flight up instead of getting up, stretching a bit, taking a few steps and going upstairs in order to provide the spine with occasional movement.

43

## Foe of discs: modern living

Great efforts have gone into the creation of kitchens where much can be accomplished in a sitting position by pressing buttons. In the kitchen of shortcuts, where everything is optimally at the same height, it is unnecessary to stretch or bend. In our modern society, the car is extensively used, and people often live in small apartments or bungalows without stairs. All these conveniences virtually eliminate daily exercise. While seeming to save people's backs, the opposite is achieved, so it becomes necessary to counter the ill-effects of these refinements by inventing exercise programs.

## The disc is a filling substance

*Bony ring with gela-tinous core*

The two most important building elements of a disc are the fibrous cartilage network and the gelatinous core it contains, the nucleus pulposus. The discs should not be imagined as compact elements similar to round, smooth vertebral bodies which are enclosed in a tight capsule and which can be removed like the links of a chain. Basically, discs are more a sort of filling substance that impedes two neighboring vertebrae from resting on top of each other in a hard and inelastic manner. Their task is to even out and weaken all forces—compression, pressure, stretching and strain—exerted on the spinal column.

At the top and bottom, the discs are fused with the neighboring vertebral bodies by a fine layer of cartilage. They are circumscribed by strong, wide, long bands which run along the whole spinal column. Since the strong tissue fibers are ring-shaped and woven like a bird's nest and since, in addition, the direction of fiber changes in each layer—i.e., it runs in the opposite direction of the neighboring fiber—this fibrous tissue plexus is quite sturdy and can be twisted and turned in almost any direction.

## The size of the body changes in the course of a day

The discs get their feathery elasticity from a gelatinous-like water cushion in their center that when tightly filled holds the connective tissue fibers in a somewhat taut position. This

44

gelatinous cushion does not have a fixed position within the disc, because it is pushed back and forth by movements of the spinal column and the resulting shifting pressure. If a person bends for a longer period of time, for example, the gelatinous cores in the area of the lumbar vertebrae gradually slip more to the rear. Where there is lordosis (curvature of the spine forward), they are increasingly pushed forward. The exertion of pressure during the course of a day causes so much fluid to be pressed out that a person is 3/4 to 1 inch shorter at night than in the morning. This is equalized again during the night, because the discs recuperate while lying down and the gelatinous cores refill with nutritive fluid. This is an important reason why lying flat is a healthy position—all discs are compelled to ''pull,'' which heightens their suction capacity. The more elevated the upper part of the body is in bed, the greater the pressure on the discs and the more difficult the exchange of matter becomes, hence the more difficult its nourishment.

*We are one inch smaller at night*

### Slipped discs and age

The aging process is accompanied by loss of fluid in the gelatinous cores of the disc tissue. The tissue eventually dries up, as can be observed by the fact that a person of 80 is 2 to 3

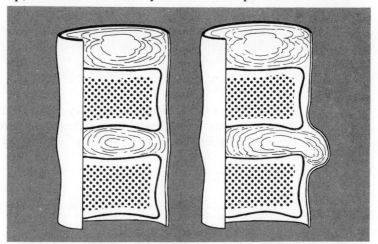

*Cross section of vertebral bodies and discs. Left:* intact disc substance. *Right:* disc substance that is arching out into the spinal canal and pressing on a nerve.

inches shorter than in youth. In addition, the disc mass, which is not contained in a firm covering, can become crumbly and break due to age and drying out. As a result, fragments of it loosen and can penetrate into the surrounding area—i.e., they prolapse. The question of whether the gelatinous core flows out with it depends in large part on how loose the fibrous cartilage ring has become. If it is torn and creates splits, a sudden movement, lifting an object suddenly or wrongly, can press out parts of it. In any case, what happens is not that a compact disc slips out as a whole in one direction or another, but rather that smaller or larger pieces of this intervertebral substance loosens itself from the whole.

Contrary to common belief, these incidents do not occur among the elderly, but most frequently among persons between 30 and 40 years of age.

<table>
<tr><td>*Most menaced age group is between 30 and 40*</td><td>Age of Patient<br>10-19<br>20-29<br>30-39<br>40-49<br>50-59<br>60-70</td><td>Prolapse Frequency<br>2.2%<br>11.2%<br>39.2%<br>29.0%<br>14.0%<br>3.0%</td></tr>
</table>

There are several reasons for this, two of which seem logical to me. First, the various tissues of a disc do not age simultaneously. It certainly does occur that its cartilaginous fiber ring may become porous, cracked, and brittle although the central gelatinous core may still be under considerable pressure from the flow. It therefore continues to fill up during periods of rest. Understandably, it can then burst the brittle disc tissue and pour out as a result of the tear. Any sudden movement or sudden bending or jerking motion can push it out. Secondly, thirty-to-forty-year olds are particularly active and have a very intense feeling for life. Their physical and emotional pendulum swings freely and they express their emotions vigorously both mentally and physically. This is in strong contrast, however, to their available strength, to their physical and mental condition, and often also to substantial lack of training. We are not only poorly trained physically and intellectually. We are also untrained emotionally, and as a result of developments in chemistry and medicine, we are relieved of all bad moods, unpleasantness, and

*Need for movement and lack of training*

46

sleeplessness.

It is difficult to provide suggestions concerning emotional training, but it can be stated that psychic stress, conflicts, and sleepless nights are part of a normal existence. For that reason, medication should not always be used in an attempt to suppress or banish such states. The practical possibilities of sensible physical training will be discussed later (page 72).

*Normal aging of discs*

Normal aging of discs need not create a problem. Almost everyone remembers having had a tired or stiff back at some time or remembers waking up in the morning with pain in the area of the small of the back that disappeared in the course of the day. When this occurs, the discs were functionally unable to keep pace—i.e., regeneration has gotten out of step with the tempo of wear and tear. The discomfort was not great enough at such times to suggest disc damage, and the trouble subsided on its own.

# Diagnosis: Sciatica

*When the nerve roots are affected*

Whenever the loosened part of a disc blocks the way of a nerve root in the lumbar area, the nerve roots react with severe pain. Prolonged pressure can actually cause the nerve to become inflamed, because its metabolism is disturbed by a pinching of the fine capillaries in its fibrous tissue covering, and it suffers lack of oxygen. The root of the sciatic nerve is most often affected, and the result is sciatic pain, or a sciatic attack.

*Typical points of pain*

Anyone who has ever had sciatica is familiar with the route of the sciatic nerve. Typical pain points are: at the side of the sacrum on the back of the pelvis; in the middle of the buttocks at the roundest part of the curve where the muscle package can be palpated through the bony proturberance; on the back side of the thigh down along the outer side to the knee and down the calf to the outer ankle. Sometimes the pain is felt only in the ankle and not along the complete route.

**What conservative treatment can accomplish**

Sciatic pain ranges from a quiet ringing that is more suspected than felt, to a tickling and numbness in certain toes, to motor

47

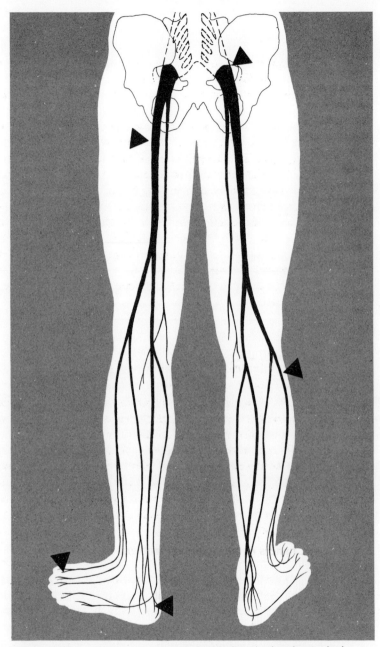

*Course of the sciatic nerve (nervus ischiadicus),* showing typical locations of pain. Pressure on this nerve can provoke sensory disturbances (feeling of numbness, piercing pain, burning sensation). In severe cases it reacts with motoric disturbances that can lead to paralysis.

disturbance, muscle weakness, or to a total collapse of muscles while standing or walking. Sciatic pain responds to traction, heat, careful massage of the fibers, and special sciatic exercises. Exercises are particularly effective in treating cases caused primarily by irritation and inflammation. When the swelling of the inflamed irritation in the root area of the nerve diminishes, pressure is relieved. Like pain caused by slipped discs, it is altogether possible that sciatic pain can be eliminated by conservative measures. Not every case involving a slipped disc requires surgery, as is assumed. Traction can often pull a disc back into place and empty it.

### The necessity of surgery

Discs that slip forward in the direction of the abdominal area rarely present a problem and in fact rarely occur, because they are suspended by a strong band which runs along the front side of the vertebrae. Slips toward the lower middle of the back occur mostly after 60 or 70 years of age and similarly can cause a longitudinal ligament that runs in this area to bulge into the vertebral canal. This usually causes only a dull pain in the small of the back. In contrast, it is very painful when disc material breaks up and slips out somewhat more toward the side but also toward the back into the nerves' exit openings through which nerve roots also pass. With motoric casualties (i.e., manifestations of paralysis) or severe uncontrollable pain, surgery is indicated immediately before the nerve becomes damaged. For these reasons, about 11% of all disc occurrences require surgical treatment.

*Disc material*
*breaks up*

### Chances of curing a disc problem

For many persons with disc problems who have had either incidents or surgery, a wider complex of questions is of great importance: what are the consequences of such a condition? Can a slipped disc incident recur? How stable is the back after a lumbar attack, sciatic irritation, or even after disc surgery?

Let us assume at the outset that a sciatic pain, a lumbago attack, or a severe pain in the small of the back really is caused by material that has crumbled out of a brittle and fragile disc. We see in practice that the danger of recurrence paradoxically

*Danger of*
*recurrence*

diminished with the intensity of the wear and tear of the disc. This is because disc tissue is not reproduced and eventually disappears. What is seen on an x-ray is a narrowing of the intervertebral space. Consequently, the connection of the vertebrae becomes tighter and less elastic, there is less room for movement between the vertebrae, and fewer irritations are possible. The process can calm down on its own, even inflamed swelling may subside, and the tension of the tissue may diminish, and when this occurs, the pain also abates.

### The formation of disc scars

Dead disc tissue undergoes change like a scar that covers over and tightens up an injury, although it cannot take over the specific functions of an organ. A scar in the heart muscle, for example, consists of fibrous tissue and not of heart muscle cells. It lacks the capacities of conduction and contraction that cells have. A scar on the liver has a cementing function but cannot participate in liver metabolism. A disc scar consists of a fibrous tissue remnant. It has no specific function, is inelastic and lacks the gelatinous water pillow. The scar, however, is stronger than the tissue fragments were before.

### Preventive stiffening

Preventive stiffening has a calming effect. Many persons are surprisingly inflexible in the small of the back; if they bend forward, this movement occurs in effect through a snap in the hip joint and a curve in the chest and neck vertebrae, while nothing moves in the lumbar area. By moving in this protective manner, they experience no pain at all. On the contrary, their backs are astonishingly efficient, and they can even do heavy physical work without pain. In such cases, no attempt should be made to force mobilization of this area by any of the means now available. This stiffening process should simply be considered one of the body's self-protective measures and as the final, although incomplete, stage of healing.

*The body's own protective measures*

Discs that have been operated on rarely cause a problem again in the same area. First, because there is no longer any disc material there that can prolapse and also because the neighboring vertebrae has been blocked by the operation. This part of the spine has gained significant stability. Secondly, each spinal column usually has only one such acutely weak point, mostly the result of a functional problem. For this reason, it is important that the total musculature be properly trained. The patient should also be made aware of his general physical capacity and how much the back can be taxed. There should also be instruction in moving back muscles and in lifting and carrying objects safely and the correct physiological use of the discs and back muscles. Attempts at training without proper instruction often omit consideration of the overall importance of the abdominal muscles, which both support and unburden the back muscles. These muscles are under-developed among persons who sit while working, because in this position the abdominal muscles are relaxed and hardly used, with the result that the back must provide all the support.

### Sciatica leads to sensitivity

*Dress warmly or condition the body?*

Anyone who has had a sciatic problem knows that a sciatic attack can last a long time, that it can occur within a span of weeks or months and then almost disappear, but that it has a way of settling in. As a result, it is possible to become so oversensitive in this area that every breath of air becomes suspect of causing pain. Knowing no other precaution, sciatic victims resort to overdressing, even to the point of wearing angora underwear. A systematic turnabout in the direction of conditioning is needed. How, where, and when to do this will be discussed later under the heading of self-help *(page 80)* at the end of the book.

# Diagnosis: Pain in the Small of the Back

### Small of the back pain among women

Pains that are felt in the small of the back but originate elsewhere are typical among women. "Among 10 women who

51

visit a gynecologist, 4 complain of pain in the small of the back, 4 others upon questioning make the same complaint, and only 2 women have no complaint"(Martius). Such pains in the area of the small of the back are gynecological in origin and so common I wish to mention the syndrome here. They often respond well to gymnastics, baths, and massages, especially to massages of the fibrous tissue.

*Pain in the small of the back related to menstruation*

Many such pains are cyclic or periodic and are related to the menstrual cycle. Their origin is in the greater emotional instability resulting in pain sensitivity caused by menstruation rather than from any organic disturbance.

It should be mentioned in this context that a change in the position of the uterus, which can be bent toward the rear (*retroflexio uteri*), or dropped, can be the cause of complaint, especially among women who have had several children. This constant pull on the inner organs, which are all anchored by bands and fibrous tissue to the bony pelvis, can start at the peritoneal cavity and irritate the sacral area. Tissue changes resulting from scarring—as can be found after an inflammation or in the area of the appendix, for example,—can irritate the small of the back area due to the pull of shrinking scar tissue. These pains can radiate into the lumbar vertebral area.

Many of these complaints can have predominantly emotional components without any detectable organic involvement. There are consequently approximately 20 different terms for this syndrome that is so difficult to localize. *Pelvephia vegetativa,* or pelvic problems having their origin in the autonomic nervous system, were so named by a gynecologist (Gauss) because medically no other description fits. The gynecologist, August Mayer, speaks especially of younger women who more frequently suffer from pains in the small of the back as "women who are fated to be ill." After menopause these complaints no longer occur, as the so-called fate has already been decided.

*Pain in the small of the back related to emotional stress*

Pain in the small of the back is often misdiagnosed as being of orthopedic origin and the patient is then sent for physiotherapy. Massages and supervised exercise help to improve circulation and relax the tense tissues. The most important part of the treatment is, however, a discussion with the patient. Talking can air a marital conflict or a lack of self-confidence and can help release emotional tension. Intense sports activity and exercise are the most effective form of treatment for this kind of pain.

Kidney problems—inflammations or tumors—can also cause

discomfort in the small of the back. Occasionally a floating kidney can also cause pain in this area.

**A problem for the small of the back: overweight**

More frequent and important is the problem of overweight. It is the back that feels the weight of a large stomach. The resulting pull on the spinal column and back muscles is enormous when the abdominal muscles, simply as a result of permanent overstretching, can no longer support the weight of the stomach. The stomach then "hangs" only from the back and strains the back musculature and lumbar vertebrae beyond their capacity.

*Concave small of the back and the stomach*

The small of the back must try to balance this overweight by creating extreme lordosis (curvature of the spine forward). This often causes the back muscles in the region to develop cords the size of an arm. The vertebrae and their spinal processes are then in a deep groove between these cords and can hardly still be palpated. In addition, even the nourishment of discs depends on weight. Discs that must support overweight are constantly burdened and under pressure. Weight is on them even in a resting position, dangerously impairing their chance of regeneration.

# Diagnosis: Rounded Back

*Causes of weak posture*

Many parents feel that a round back in children is the result of relaxed, careless posture, a poor habit that can be corrected by strict pedagogical measures. However, poor posture in most cases is organic in origin, because a tired back also indicates a poor relation between the existing and needed strength. Supportive tissue can qualitatively be highly or poorly developed. This weakness either has inherited biological reasons or is conditioned by environmental factors such as urban living.

*Damage caused by the environment*

Such factors include the strain of living in air polluted from car exhausts, constant walking on cement that overtaxes the spinal column, lack of movement both during and after school, and too much sitting both in school and over homework.

We have already mentioned that sitting places the greatest strain on the discs *(page 43)*. We must add that disc tissue, like other body and cell tissue, is continually replaced, which means

53

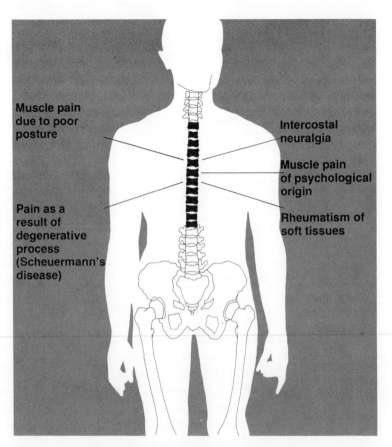

**Muscle pain due to poor posture**

**Intercostal neuralgia**

**Muscle pain of psychological origin**

**Pain as a result of degenerative process (Scheuermann's disease)**

**Rheumatism of soft tissues**

*Thoracic vertebral column.* Source of all disturbances and morbid diseases of the thoracic vertebral column. The illustration shows the origin of specific complaints.

there is an ongoing process of intercellular decomposition and regeneration. This deterioration is part of the normal life process and has nothing to do with disc wear and tear. With the exception of the nerve cells of the central nervous system, no cell attains the age of the person in whose body it is found. According to Kraemer, the length of time a disc is capable of providing support—i.e., the time in which its cells are renewed—is only a few weeks. If disc metabolism is impeded, the body produces increasingly inferior disc tissue instead of healthy tissue. Therefore, if children are physically too burdened and cannot move about enough for their discs to be adequately trained in the necessary change from pressure and pull, from strain and relaxation, the result is weakness both in the capacity and quality of their supporting tissue—i.e., in the spinal column and discs. A rounded back is the result.

*Curvature of the spinal column*

How a person sits is as important as the duration of time spent sitting. In a classroom of children age twelve and thirteen, some are in stature already men and cannot fix their six-foot frames into school desks. They must put an extra curve in the chest region of the spinal column even to be able to read from a book. Often tall persons prefer to recline in low seating rather than to sit properly. By doing so, two-thirds of the body is in a horizontal position, and only one-third upright. The curve necessary to achieve this position is in the vicinity of the upper thoracic part of the spine, which is where they either have a hump or where it is starting to form. Back fatigue due to weakness of tissue is not only a bad habit but a problem to be countered first medically and then pedagogically. In addition,

*Target area for psychological stress*

this is precisely the area that reacts to and shows psychological stress. A hunched back can still be fairly well corrected at an early age by stretching and strengthening exercises. A hunched back in an adult gradually becomes stiff and requires extra strength to keep it upright, especially since the muscles have adjusted to this condition. The back muscles become inactive and weak in the area between the shoulder blades. Because the muscles are under latent tension from being used for the purpose of pulling the shoulders back and because the muscles and tendons around the front of the armpit pull the shoulders forward, the muscles shrivel up and in time become shorter. As a consequence, hanging from the arms—as on a gym bar, for example—becomes painful. This condition can be helped through slow, systematic stretching. Such exercises must, however, always be accompanied by strengthening exercises for the whole back.

# Diagnosis: "Scheurmann's" Disease, or Juvenile Kyphosis

If a young man lies down in a prone position without being able to flatten his hunched back, and if the hump is even more

*An illness
that occurs
during
puberty*

noticeable than in standing, then he probably suffered during puberty from ''Scheurmann's Disease,'' so named after its discoverer. The course of this disease is hardly noted by persons in the vicinity or even by the patient himself. The starting point of these changes, which occur mainly in the lower section of the thoracic part of the spine and usually among young males, are degenerative changes in the vertebral bodies whose upper plates change in structure and soften. They increasingly lose their load-bearing capacity, resulting in partial fractures and the entry of disc material into the vertebrae. This interspersion of intervertebral material, which later usually calcifies (named for

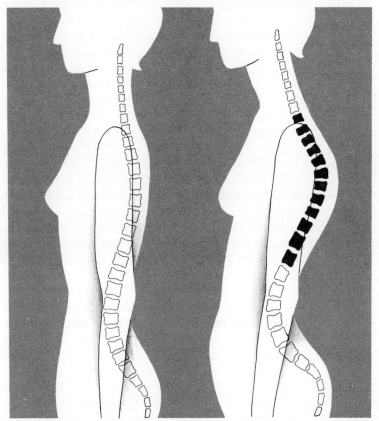

*Final stage of Scheurmann's disease that was not treated in time. Left:* physiological curvature is healthy, stretched spinal column. *Right:* Scheurmann round back with compensatory hollow in the small of the back and wedge-shaped, flattened vertebral bodies in the area of the historic vertebral column.

56

its discoverer and termed *Schmorl's knots*) and is visible on the x-ray of an adult, is often the only indication of the process that

*Early corrective measures necessary*

occurred during puberty. If the condition is noted early, it can be impeded through exercise, or if necessary, by the use of a cast while sleeping. If this process in the spinal column is undetected, such degeneratively changed vertebrae can break under strain. Depending on the amount of pressure exerted, they become wedge-shaped, almost triangular when viewed from the side. A rounding of the back then becomes organically fixed, stiffens, and cannot be straightened later.

As these changes of the vertebrae occur only during puberty, it is assumed that there is some hormonal influence. This syndrome is usually found among tall children who grew extremely rapidly or among those who had to do heavy physical labor during their development; hence the more familiar designation of the disease, "Apprentice Kyphosis." (*kyphosis* is a bending of the spine toward the rear; *lordosis*, a bending toward the front; *scoliosis*, a bending toward the side.) This type of vertebral change is extremely rare among girls, although cases do occur.

# Diagosis: Intercostal Neuralgia

Disc problems rarely occur in the area of the thoracic vertebrae. There are two reasons for this. First, since the ribs are attached in front to the chest bone, this area of the spine moves much less than that of the lumbar area. Secondly, the nerves' exit points are relatively large in comparison with the thin intercostal nerves (the nerves between the ribs) that leave the spinal column at this level. Therefore the danger of pinching a nerve root is greatly lessened. Irritations of the intercostal nerves do occur, however, and are called neuralgias. They are caused by an early aging process in the cartilage-bone-tissue of the vertebrae (both

*Irritations of the intercostal nerves*

in the vertebral bodies and the small vertebral joints) and are a form of osteochondrosis (see page 58). This can also cause the vertebrae to fuse together and can cause constriction of the nerve root, congestion, and metabolic disturbance of the fibrous tissue coverings. Irritation and pain are the result.

Many patients with intercostal neuralgia go to a doctor, imagining they are suffering from heart pain. They often initially

57

question the accuracy of the doctor's diagnosis and the necessity of the physiotherapeutic treatment then prescribed. The stabbing pains in the heart area are the same as those imagined from real heart pain, so it is difficult for the patient to understand that this is an orthopedic problem in the area of the thoracic vertebrae. This is due to the fact that these intercostal nerves also have fibrous connections to vegetative nerves, particularly to those that reach such internal organs as the heart. The result can be a reflex short circuit, which explains how root irritation of an intercostal nerve can actually simulate pain in the area of the heart.

Intercostal neuralgias are subjectively so disagreeable because every breath produces a stabbing pain. The victim then scarcely dares to breathe assuming the pleura to be involved also. Treating the back with warmth, massage of the fibrous tissue, careful mobilization of the chest, and even the use of medication in acute stages usually improve the condition.

# Diagnosis: Osteochondrosis

Osteochondrosis is a degenerative rather than an inflammatory change of the cartilage-bone-tissue. It can develop on any bone-cartilage transition, even where the articular surfaces glide over each other. A knee joint arthrosis, called *arthrosis deformans* because in advanced cases it can cause bizarre deformities of the knee, is in a sense actually an osteochondrosis. So, too, is the wearing-out of the hip joint and coxarthrose, which is know as *arthrosis deformans* of the hip

joint. The cartilage-bone changes present here are the same at all joints, whether on one as large as the hip joint or as small as the vertebral joint. The cartilage layer that covers the surfaces of the joint and makes it capable of gliding becomes more fibrous, in part deteriorates, and is replaced by bony ridges and growths. As a result, the joint crevice gradually contracts and the surfaces of the joint lose their ability to glide over each other. This condition is a mechanical source of pain. In addition, tension usually develops in the joint capsule, which fills with fluid. The body always reacts to such chronically inflamed processes as occur in joint changes by secreting additional fluid. If bacteria are not originally responsible for the irritation, as is the case in

58

acute joint rheumatism, then such effusion from the joint consists of clear tissue fluid. There is also usually a sympathetic reaction by the surrounding musculature of such an irritated joint. Both the attempt to block out the pain by keeping the joint immobile—i.e., by a heightened defense reaction—and the immediate pull of tension on the joint capsule and the surrounding tissue only heighten the irritation. This is one of the instances when the defense mechanism of the body works to its disadvantage. This occurs frequently in heart-circulatory proc-esses.

# Diagnosis: CVC Syndrome

The comprehensive term for a specific complex of symptoms in

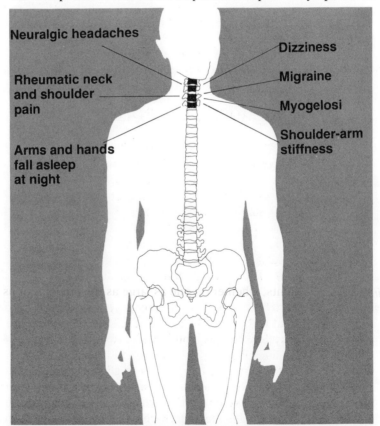

Neuralgic headaches

Dizziness

Rheumatic neck
and shoulder
pain

Migraine

Myogelosi

Shoulder-arm
stiffness

Arms and hands
fall asleep
at night

*Cervical vertebral column.* Area of the cervical vertebral column with CVC syndrome showing the possible consequences of osteochondrotic changes.

the area of the lumbar vertebral column is abbreviated LVC. Similarly, the term for problems in the area of the cervical vertebral column is CVC syndrome. The changes, especially the early beginnings of wear and tear of the cartilage and bones in the neck area, resemble those of the lumbar vertebral area. The flexibility of the cervical vertebral area is extremely great in all directions. It carries the head, which is the center and seat of our life-supporting sense organs. Fundamental security reasons require the quickest possible perception of sense impressions, so the functioning of the CVC is very important; its condition, like other sections of the spine, is closely tied to its particular musculature, the neck and throat musculature.

### Whiplash and lumbago in the area of the cervical vertebral column

*Effects on the throat and neck muscles*

Anyone who has had a lumbago attack, a sudden muscle cramp in the area of the throat-neck muscles, or a whiplash caused by one car colliding with another from the rear, causing the person to feel massive strain in this area of the neck muscle,

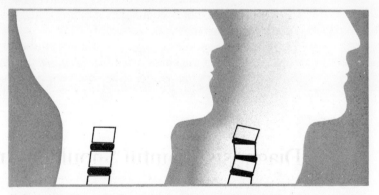

*Left:* a normal cervical vertebral column with pronounced intercertebral discs. *Right:* a worn cervical vertebral column showing intervertebral discs that have become markedly thinner.

is familiar with the resulting handicap. It is no longer possible to turn one's head. Instead turns must be carefully made by the

60

whole body, it is no longer possible to twist around in changing directions, and in order to sleep the head must be set down with extreme care.

Disc wear and tear and degenerative changes of the vertebral bodies and joints do occur in the throat area. Such processes often begin between twenty and thirty years of age. They usually remain dormant for a long time, then suddenly begin to reach consciousness through a quick backward movement of the head, a strong draft from riding in a car with an open window, or from a massive jolt of the vertebral column caused by stepping into emptiness instead of onto a step.

*A cold results in lumbago*

Slipped discs, however, are very rare in the cervical vertebral area, as the discs between the vertebrae of the neck area are better anchored by bony protuberances than those between the lumbar vertebrae. Nerves coming from the cervical part of the medulla can nonetheless become pinched due to osteochondrotically changed vertebrae which cause constriction of the exit points of the nerves. Even the great artery of the neck, the *a. vertebralis*, which runs upward in a canal formed by transverse processes of the cervical vertebrae along the side of the neck to the occipital foramen, can be constricted by such osteochondrotic changes. The same is true of a nerve network containing vegetative fibers that accompanies it. This particular nerve network is called the *plexus vertebralis*.

*Pinched nerve*

As a result of all these processes, the nerve roots in this area, which come from the spinal cord, can also become irritated. Here, as in other areas of the spinal column, the response is the same—pain.

# Diagnosis: Painful Shoulder-Arm Stiffness

In the area of the neck, the possibilities for disturbed nerves to cause irritation by pressure are especially varied. The "projection fields" of pain are also particularly great. Such referred pain may be felt as migraine attacks and neuralgic headaches that extend from the back of the head to the brow like a metal ring around the head or as radiating pains in the shoulder-arm area. There is a typical, delineated syndrome for this area: painful

61

shoulder-arm stiffness or *periarthritis humero-scapularis*.

Although this term sounds pompous, it accurately designates the points attacked and the affected area. Periarthritis means that inflammatory changes around the joint area are occurring—in this case, the shoulder joint—and the upper arm (the humerus) and the shoulder blade (scapula) are affected.

An early alarm signal is nightly numbness of the hands and arms. This manifestation is actually found in all degenerative changes in the area of the neck vertebrae and generally shows that circulation is no longer functioning properly. It is caused by muscle cramping that results in changes in the cervical vertebral column itself and in the musculature of this area.

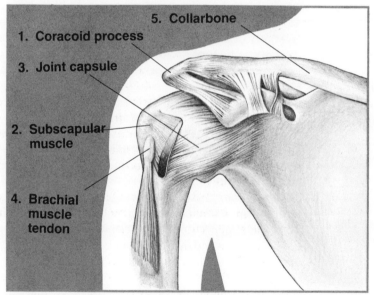

*Illustration of the joint capsule and all bones and muscles involved in shoulder-arm stiffness.*
Musculus subscapularis (2) enters the joint capsule at this point, the shoulder connection, which is the main location of pain resulting from shoulder-arm stiffness. This muscle pulls the arm toward the rear and turns it toward the inside (apron string muscle). Tendon of the musculus biceps brachii (4), the brachial muscle. Where there is shoulder-arm stiffness, it becomes painful and brittle; calcium deposits can form, and it can tear.

These are merely early symptoms. The actual shoulder-arm stiffness, the final result of these degenerative changes in the shoulder-arm area, is in its symptomatology quite unmistakeable and extremely painful.

The shoulder-arm stiffness described by those affected is often so typical that it is recognizable from the mere description even before palpating the tensed neck muscles and the widespread condition of myogelosis, hearing the cracking sound toward in the top of the shoulder, and even before examining x-rays of the patient. Any jolting motion of the arm is painful, especially a forward thrusting motion, and it is almost impossible to make the apronstring movement in which the arms move back and inward simultaneously. Lifting an arm to the side is often difficult because of radiating pain that may extend to the fingers. Pressure on the top of the front shoulder, which cracks during movement, is also painful.

*Grating in the shoulder cap*

At this point in the flexible shoulder-arm connection involving the bony continuations of the shoulder blade, collar bone, and head of the upper arm, there are muscles and tendons that radiate into the joint capsule and periosteum. If these muscles are subjected for longer periods of time to heightened tension, they contribute significantly to irritating the tissue surrounding the point by pulling on the periosteum, which is acutely sensitive to pain. Such a painful arm is naturally moved little. Once limitation of movement has occurred, it often presents the greatest therapeutic problem.

*Pain sensitivity of the periosteum*

The tendons, tissues of the organism having extremely weak metabolism, are damaged from being subject to pulling tension. Their metabolic state thus deteriorates further. They become brittle and cracked and lose elasticity as a result of calcium deposits. Consequently, in advanced cases a torn tendon can result. With the exception of a torn tendon, which requires surgical treatment, the other periarthritic changes are to a large extent reversible. This means that they can recede, and such a joint can even become free of pain and flexible again. Treatment, however, should begin before mechanical impairment of movement has occurred. The joint capsule, which is particularly broad here in order to provide the greatest radius of arm movement, should not be permitted to become conglutenated and ultimately deformed. Such a development can occur very rapidly at the shoulder joint, because the capsule forms larger folds under the shoulder when the arms hang down. These folds will conglutinate or adhere as soon as they are no longer "unfolded."

*Inhibited movement of the shoulder joint*

63

Nothing can be done about degenerative cartilage-bone changes, osteochonrosis of the lumbar vertebral column also cannot be changed. It is possible, however, to prevent muscle tension, to help maintain flexibility of the cervical vertebrae and take measures to ensure balanced movement. This is especially important for people whose work involves much sitting, necessitates holding the neck and shoulders in a cramped position, or where one-sided work is involved—as, for example, secretaries, dentists, and persons working at sewing machines. Even farmers engaged in an allegedly healthy occupation are affected. The mechanization of agriculture has even made farming a hazardous occupation. The vibration places a strain on the spinal column, the exhaust fumes damage the lungs, and the necessity of turning the whole body around to check on and control the apparatus being pulled behind the tractor produces muscle strain.

# Diagnosis: Disturbances of the Cerebral Blood Supply

*Lack of blood supply to the brain*

The great artery, the *arteria vertebralis*, runs through a bony canal formed by transverse processes of the cervical vertebrae. As a result of its direction, it is as prone to disturbance by changes of the cervical vertebrae as the *plexus vertebralis*, a vegetative nerve network accompanying it. Any impairment of the blood flow in this vessel, especially due to osteochondrotic bone swelling and clasping, can result in defective circulation to the brain and attacks of dizziness. This is very dangerous to car drivers, persons who work at machines, surgeons, pilots, or to persons in any occupation requiring a high degree of concentration.

The role of the neck musculature, as the main target area of muscular tension resulting from mechanical strain and mental and emotional stress, has already been discussed in detail (page 23).

In concluding our discussion of the whole area of the spinal column, it is still necessary to discuss numerous disturbances that can occur at particular points or in all the areas of the back as a functioning unit. These disturbances involve back complaints due to postural deviation and include musculature, ligaments, the pelvis, the ribs, breathing and the neck.

# Diagnosis: Postural Damage

*Balance through muscular equilibrium*

A healthy spinal column that has normal posture wears well to a large extent as a result of its slight curves. It is capable of balancing itself out by the feathery interplay of ligaments, the cartilaginous intervertebral discs, and the muscle covering that catches and balances out each movement. If the muscular balance is intact, body symmetry is completely assured, so the organism requires a minimum of strength to balance out such a tall column as the human body on such an extraordinarily small base as the feet. The work of the musculature primarily consists of constant tension and release, of movement and stopping. Each stimulus is answered with a counterreaction, each impulse is echoed and releases the muscular counter-impulse in its muscular counterpart. The body always tries to keep the forces in balance, because every disturbance in this labile balance means an increased burden and necessitates additional expenditure and use of strength and energy.

### Disturbances in the balance of strength and body symmetry

*Equilibrium of the body*

The reason a person who limps tires more quickly is not because a weak leg fails, but because healthy muscles must work harder. An *arthrosis deformans* of a knee joint mainly strains the healthy leg, whose hip joint tries to compensate for the imbalance. Sitting mainly causes pain in the back because in this position the back lacks the muscular support of the abdominal muscles and must provide unaided the supportive work intended for its counterpart (the chest and abdominal musculature). Thus every muscular weakness requires additional exertion by another muscle—i.e., every functional exception produces an echo. Understanding the possible effect of changes within the body's total equilibrium requires imagining the physiological strength necessary for maintaining an optimally energy-saving posture.

65

### The transition from four legs to two

Balancing on four legs, or on four support points, is much easier and energy-saving than upright walking. This is common knowledge requiring no further explanation. In making the transition, though, from this kind of movement to upright

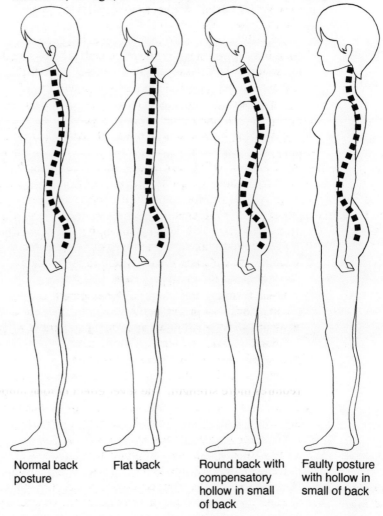

Normal back posture

Flat back

Round back with compensatory hollow in small of back

Faulty posture with hollow in small of back

Comparisons between normal body posture (*left*) and the most frequent postural deviations

walking, which changes must be made? And what must be adjusted to make an upright gait energy-saving? What happens in standing and walking?

*The anatomical transition*

A child just at the crawling stage making its first attempts at standing and walking clearly illustrates the period of anatomical transition. It is mainly possible by observing where difficulties in equilibrium occur, witnessing the striving for balance, and noting where and why a child falls.

Initially a small child still makes a big bend in the hips while standing. Also, the axis around which all movements of the torso occur still passes through the hip joint. If the child loses its balance, it bends at the hip and sits down. In order to compensate for this emphasis on hip-bending, a strong lumbar lordosis (bending to the front) is needed—i.e., it needs a hollow small of the back and above it a relatively flat back. The neck and its curvature are scarcely involved yet. A broad support base is needed for bearing this small body, which is difficult to balance, whose weight is unevenly distributed, and whose center of gravity is still too much to the rear. For these reasons, a child

*The toddler's posture*

stands straddle-legged; even walking still takes place in the transverse axis and, lacking strength of step, he stomps instead. Added height makes balancing easier—the spinal column becomes flexible and the body acquires the pattern for moving the feet—and the child is then able to walk.

Basic forms of this postural development can still be found among adults—a pronounced lumbar lordosis, a hollow small of the back and the resulting protruding abdomen, a flat back, remnants of early patterns of movement such as stomping, a heavy gait, and a too erect back posture. As the size of the body increases, such postural deviation becomes more difficult and requires more strength. The lever effect of long limbs on the torso is felt, the torso musculature itself must span larger areas, and the demand for balanced movement increases.

*What influences standing and walking*

Even the fulcrum around which the adult body's long axis moves has been shifted. An important axis now goes through the ankle. The bending angle in the ankle joint determines the position toward the front or toward the rear in standing and walking. Simultaneously it determines the necessary muscular balance and the musculature's expenditure of energy. Going up and down an incline changes this bending angle just as does the heel height of a shoe. Any impairment of movement or a stiffening of this joint makes walking choppy and robs it of its

67

flow. In addition, it impairs the possibility of dividing body weight between the length of step taken by each leg and of continuing to move from one foot to the other without interruption. This also strains other muscle groups, which in turn must work harder, and produces an imbalance of muscle strain.

The toddler's strongly tilted pelvis becomes straight in a normally developed adult, and the hip joint has also stretched. The lumbar lordosis is less pronounced and is mainly taken up by the slight convexity of the thoracic vertebral column, which gently passes into the neck lordosis. The interplay of these three normal physiological curvatures produces the feathery elasticity of the spinal column. These curvatures prevent the head from jolting and distribute the changing pressure on the system of intervertebral discs. A flat back and very upright position of the spinal column make it react more severely to pressure; a round back reacts more severely to pull. A hollow small of the back creates increased cutting forces between the rigid sacrum and the flexible lumbar vertebrae. Such postural deviations result in greater wear of the bones, cartilage, and tendons.

*Origin of equilibrium problems*

Such postural deviations affect the muscles even more severely. Back muscles that must span a round back are stretched beyond capacity. The front chest muscles become shorter because the shoulders are being pulled forward, which makes pulling them back more difficult. The torso no longer supports itself, and straightening it up requires strength. The back muscles involved become latently tense, their tone heightens, they tire, and then the back hurts. An extremely hollow small of the back causes the abdominal muscles to become overstretched, and the hip flexors shortened. This makes lifting the pelvis more difficult, the extensors of the back become hard strands, they tire, and the result is back pain. Deviations of balance are still more decisive in a lateral direction. A unilateral body asymmetry, for example, becomes a scoliosis, which is a lateral curvature of the spinal column.

All muscles and muscle groups in the body are paired. This means that each half of the body has its corresponding muscles on the opposite side. Every movement that occurs without friction depends upon balance and upon the capacity of each side to work synchronically and synergetically—i.e., with the same energy. If this symmetry is disturbed, one of the muscle groups must work harder to equalize the lack of strength of the other side and take over its work load. Consequently, it tires more quickly, the muscle tone is heightened, and the back hurts.

Many persons have a slight asymmetry of the back caused by a weak lateral curvature—i.e., scoliosis of the spinal column—but they are unaware of it and notice no impairment of function. Among the previously mentioned 85% of all persons having postural anomalies, a large number are such slight cases of scoliosis.

Even a slight change in the symmetry of the supportive apparatus is accompanied by a corresponding shift of muscular balance. This has no effect on normal use of a back that has sufficient alternation between tension and relaxation, adequate oxygen, and movement. But where there is monotonous strain caused from long periods of standing, bending, or sitting, the muscular imbalance will result in the muscularly stronger side's helping the weaker side by taking over its work load. That will be the side of the back that will soon manifest myogelosis, hard tendons, and painful cramps of the overworked musculature. Shoulder-arm stiffness, dislocated discs, muscle pain in the neck, and neuralgic headaches will also result from such imbalance.

**Cause of postural deviation**

There are many reasons involved in postural deviations that affect the supporting apparatus: the basic quality of the tissue, way of life, the degree of strain on the back, the way of moving, proper or insufficient diet. Illnesses and injuries in particular are often responsible for postural deviation. Even the shortening of a leg by less than half an inch as the result of a broken bone ultimately reacts negatively on the equilibrium. A hip joint can manifest wear and tear early. It can affect the spinal column in the form of a tipped pelvis and become noticeable by the resulting asymmetry of the musculature. A raised shoe usually helps in such cases. But the problem of balancing a muscle weakened from paralysis, a too-flattened angle of a fracture of the neck of the femur, a stiffened knee joint, or a curved spinal column present enormous problems of equilibrium. All such problems result in strain registered in the muscles and joints. Ultimately their initial cause is irrelevant. The course of a postural deviation—whether it primarily affects the supportive apparatus by a constitutional weakness in the tissues and tendons, subsequently causing muscle imbalance, or whether the chain reaction began with a weakened muscle that curved the spine because of unequal muscle pull—is not so important for therapy. What is much more relevant is to attempt to correct the deviation and, wherever possible, to prevent it.

What is important in the many small postural weaknesses and deviations, regardless of their course, is the attainment of muscle quality. The following are effective preventive measures: the prevention of loss of muscle strength by early and consistent muscle training, by an adequate supply of oxygen obtained by much outdoor exercise, frequent alternation between tension and release of muscles even during work. Weight is also important, because overweight considerably worsens postural weakness.

*Prevention through training*

70

# 4. Correct Breathing

## Its Value for the Organism

A diagnosis of faulty or inadequate breathing is not often made, even though it could apply to every second patient seeking physiotherapy treatment for a back or spinal column syndrome and should be treated. Proper breathing necessitates mobilization of the chest cavity, resulting in improved blood supply to the tissues and in relaxation.

*Proper breathing*

Breathing is one of the most fundamental life processes. To understand the importance of intensive breathing and to provide motivation for the observation and improvement of your own breathing, I wish to point out some of the interrelationships of the physiology of breathing.

### The breathing mechanism

The breathing mechanism is especially important in any consideration of back problems, because it is closely tied to body posture and the upright position of the spinal column. It is also very dependent on the elasticity of the rather short muscles of the thorax, or the chest cavity. Basically, these muscles function statically. Inhaling is an active event that results in the enlargement of the inner chest cavity. The ribs are flexibly connected to the spinal column and run from the spine diagonally toward the front. The increase in the volume of the

71

chest cavity thus occurs through a simple tilting turn of the ribs in these small dorsal vertebral joints. At the moment of inhaling they are lifted and almost horizontal. This can easily be felt by placing the hands lightly on the side of the chest cavity. Anyone who has ever popped a button on a tight shirt knows that the lower edge of the ribs expands and is the part that is raised highest. The button popped was not in the upper chest area but rather one over the abdominal area, where the lower breathing space is optimally enlarged.

*What con-*
*stricts the*
*breathing*
*area*

If we try to visualize the breathing mechanism, we can see how severely postural deviations affect breathing. The curved spinal column of a rounded back restricts the breathing space; a spinal column bent to the side pushes the ribs out on one side but pulls them in on the other and impairs breathing significantly; and cramped, adhered back muscles that virtually wall in the chest cavity can bring the sensitive act of breathing mechanically almost to a halt.

The lungs themselves are passively affected, since they are covered all over by a skin, or pleura. The chest wall is also covered with pleura on the inside. These two coverings are held tight and yet are moveably tied together by a layer of fluid similar to a wet, airtight, closed plastic bag. Their surfaces shift freely over each other but cannot be separated. If the inner chest cavity expands (the thoracic area), the lung is expanded with it. The lung is then stretched and unfolded and in this manner compelled to suck in air. Muscles used in breathing include the diaphragm and the small in-between rib muscles, so if contraction of the breathing muscle diminishes, the thorax again contracts due to its elastic components. The lungs are involved in this process, so the air streams out again. How much the inner chest area can expand depends on the quality of the muscles necessarily involved, the flexibility of the ribs, the elasticity of the tendons and joints, and especially on body posture and the erectness of the spinal column.

*Breathing*
*muscles*
*expand the*
*thoracic area*

A round back provides the ribs with a poor basis for the necessary expansion of the breathing area, because the curvature of the spinal column causes the ribs to drop down significantly. The breathing muscles are no longer able to lift the ribs into a horizontal position in order to enlarge the breathing area. The lungs are not fully unfolded and stretched and do not take in enough air; exhalation is also poor and incomplete. In this case, exhalation is more a matter of compliance by the

72

spinal column and a collapse of the entire thorax rather than, as it should be, a real contraction supported by the elasticity of the tissue in the chest cavity and lung. A stretched, erect spinal column offers optimal breathing amplitude by providing the ribs with much room for movement between diagonal and horizontal positions, permits a flexible descent into the resting position, thereby assuring complete exhalation.

What happens while breathing and its importance in relation to backaches will become clear when we recall the possible cause of muscle pain and when we take into consideration, both here and in reference to the metabolism of our discs, that lack of oxygen is the cause of all degenerative and painful conditions. Adequate supply of oxygen is linked functionally to adequate breathing.

*Circulation and breathing*

A last link in this chain of mutual dependency is the mechanism of circulation, which we shall now examine only from the perspective of blood as a means of transporting oxygen. As already explained, the quality of tissue depends on its blood supply. The blood supplied must contain sufficient oxygen, however—i.e., a sufficient number of red blood corpuscles carrying sufficient oxygen. The process of oxygen intake, the possibility of contact between blood and air, depends mainly on qualitatively good breathing.

Among the factors that assure good breathing, the following are of primary importance: the largest possible breathing volume so that enough air cells (alveoli) are opened up to permit optimal assimilation of oxygen and an elastic chest cavity to provide optimal emptying of the lungs during exhalation. Good air containing oxygen is of course vitally necessary.

Even this brief statement indicates that one of the essential conditions for functionally intact, pain-free musculature is an elastic thorax and a stimulus to breathing provided by a great deal of fresh air and movement. Conversely, the breathing

*Movement as a stimulus to breathing*

movement, if it is large enough, automatically assures a flexible thorax. It assures a kind of ongoing training for maintaining the elasticity of the chest cavity, and only a flexible chest cavity provides a pain-free back.

The same conformity is the basis for the gaseous interchange in the tissues (inner breathing or tissue breathing). Their optimal functioning requires the availability of a sufficient number of arterial capillaries for good circulation in the muscle tissue. The blood supplied must also contain enough oxygen so the stream of metabolism finds enough diffusion gradients—i.e., can take place in the cell itself. This aspect of breathing is particularly deficient in a cramped muscle that clamps off its own capillaries. Its clusters of myogelosis enlarge as a group as a result of reduced muscle metabolism, with the result that such tensed muscles cannot adequately dispose of waste. This explains the importance of intensive breathing to internal muscle metabolism.

*Breathing observed externally*

In addition, a greater need for oxygen may be caused by physical exertion and can be satisfied by deeper or more frequent breathing (number of breaths per minute) or by both. A healthy organism controls this regulating mechanism itself; a trained heart-lung system adjusts effortlessly to these demands. This is not true of someone physically out of shape who suddenly decides to participate in a 30-mile hike or is overcome by a sudden urge to be slim. His thorax has neither the elasticity nor the necessary capacity for the air needed and his circulation cannot adjust on such short notice. His heart cannot spontaneously supply blood and must try to make up this deficit by beating more frequently. The strain on the heart is enormous, and for this reason it is medically unsound for a person unaccustomed to exercise to suddenly overexert.

### Decreased tension by breathing

The last important topic concerning breathing and heightened tension of back musculature is the possibility of releasing tension by breathing. This can be done by autogenetic training. These methods will not be explained here, because much has been written on the subject, and instruction is available from many schools and doctors. However, the principle of relaxation through breathing is so important for back muscle cramping that it will be included here. It consists in an attempt to strengthen the passive aspects of exhalation by freeing oneself from the conscious activity of breathing, simply permitting breathing to occur while regarding one's own breathing rhythm as a kind of neutral observer. If some distance is achieved (as suggested by the slogan used in training, "it is breathing me"), breathing becomes slower, calmer, and deeper. The whole body then relaxes and tension decreases. This in turn reduces general tension in the autonomic nervous system and diminishes muscle tone. The feeling of heaviness and warmth with which all

74

autogenetic training begins is the result of primary muscular relaxation. This method of relaxation is important both physically and psychologically, because it can be learned and can help in daily stress situations.

### Chest breathing—abdominal breathing

Dogmatic views are often voiced concerning the question of whether chest breathing or abdominal breathing is preferable. Due to the anatomical form of the ribs, it is alleged that during inhalation the chest cavity expands more in the lower region, especially toward the sides, while the upper chest cavity is less involved in the expansion of the chest area. It stretches more toward the front instead. The diaphragm, by flattening during inhalation, expands the inner chest area downward and facilitates abdominal breathing. It is less active in chest breathing, as it arches up into the chest area during exhalation as a result of pressure exerted by the intestines.

*Breathing impeded by pressure from intestines*

Hence it is clear that abdominal breathing, by facilitating greater expansion of the chest area, is actually more effective. However, technical reasons frequently prevent its usage. Some of these reasons are tight clothing, constriction of the abdominal area while sitting—as at a school desk or during a long drive. Another common reason in the world's more affluent countries is excessive fat. Strong pressure of the intestines causes the diaphragm to shift upward and greatly impedes breathing. This also crowds the lungs and the heart and can result in severe vegetative disturbances.

What promotes abdominal breathing, what releases it and simultaneously avoids consciously forced breathing? All forms of sport activity stimulate abdominal breathing: bicycle riding, hiking, swimming, dancing, ball playing, and also running games. In these activities abdominal breathing occurs automatically in order to supply the extra oxygen needed by the muscles, because mere thoracic breathing without the intensive participation of the diaphragm would not be sufficient. The combination of playing and moving is very important in stimulating and promoting relaxation. The absence of the necessity to assert oneself or to win, to be first or best, has a refreshing and relaxing effect that also stimulates breathing. Non-competitive sport may also provide an opportunity to laugh, even at oneself,

75

whereas any sport involving competition heightens concentration and tension and brings with it the danger of cramping.

*Singing is good training for proper breathing*

The best, healthiest, and least forced form of training in proper breathing is singing. We should sing to ourselves while driving, doing housework, where and whenever possible, simply for the sheer joy of life itself. I know a heart patient who, through a combination of outdoor exercise and hearty singing, improved her heart condition and general weakness to the extent of being able to resume a full and normal life. Records and tapes have dampened our own zest for singing, and even children now hardly sing because no one sings with them. In many families, even Christmas carols are sung by choruses seen on television. Thus we leave unused this possibility of pleasant, unforced training in breathing and strengthening the thorax. We are impelled by perfection that can be bought. In this area we have lost our naiveté.

# 5. Circulation— Conditioning Training

## The Mechanisms for Improved Blood Supply

*Increasing the capacity for good circulation*

When we speak of the circulation in tissues or organs, we mean that there is an adequate supply of blood and oxygen. This depends on the diameter of the blood vessel and on the thickness of the small hair-like capillaries that supply an organ (the number of them varies depending on need). If a greater supply of blood is needed, the capacity of the separate vessels can be increased, or other blood vessels can also assist.

## The Effect of Warmth

*Improved circulation through warmth*

Warmth is a strong stimulus toward circulation. This can be clearly felt and observed in any abrupt temperature change—for example, it can be observed in winter by holding one's pale, numb hand under warm running water and noticing how rapidly the fresh red color returns, right down into the fingertips. A thorough warming always results in improved circulation. Because of the body's need to maintain a constant body

77

temperature, it makes available as many blood vessels as possible, including all the capillaries, for distributing additional warmth through the body as quickly as possible, and the area warmed becomes red.

# Nervous-reflex Blood Supply

The warming effect of circulation can be accomplished by the use of a nervous reflex—as, for example, by warming the Head's zones of an organ—thereby creating a stimulus (in this case, to affect the blood supply) that reaches the deep-lying organ.

Many important centers and nerve bundles of the vegetative nervous system, which is involved in controlling all life processes, lie in the inner pelvic area. These can also be affected externally—from the rear side of the pelvis, for example. Fibrous tissue massage is one technique which is always started on the rear side of the pelvis with the use of heat that is then well distributed from this point. If one is thoroughly frozen through on a wet November day and has cold feet, even cold knees, it is far more effective to put the small of the back against a source of warmth than to try to warm one's feet with a hot water bottle. The connection between the pelvis and feet is more intensive and faster in its effect as a result of a reflected process.

# Stretching Exercises for Muscles in Static Demand

Stretching also has a beneficial effect on circulation to the musculature. Some muscle tension is present even when the muscle is not in use. If a non-functioning muscle were cut at one end, it would shrivel up because its fibrous tissue portions surrounding the separate muscle strands and fiber bundles would shorten. Stretching is useful as a circulatory stimulus to muscles whose main function is to provide support. In these muscles it is difficult to stimulate the metabolism through a change of tension and release, because short muscle fibers are less able to

*Muscle
stretching
as a stimulus
to circulation*

78

contract. Stretching creates much tension to which the muscle responds with a stimulus to contract. Hence stretching is comparable to passive muscle activity, since no movement is involved. Nonetheless, it is followed by a recovery period during which muscle metabolism increases. This alternation between stretching and relaxation is also actually accompanied by a certain alternation in the push and pull effect on the larger blood vessels, which similarly improves circulation. The mechanical stretching stimulus relaxes the muscles and the fibrous tissue portions—i.e., the tendons and joints. This can be felt, for example, by lying on the floor with arms raised like a half-moon until the entire chest and sides are stretched. If one again lies down after several minutes, one can notice that the whole area that was stretched has become looser, warm, and light. An alternation between tension and relaxation, or muscle activity, has a greater effect on the blood flow to muscles that have a large action radius.

# Isometric Exercises

*Effectiveness or ineffectiveness of an exercise*

Isometric muscle exercises are widely used today for releasing tension. To understand their popularity and to be able to distinguish between effective and ineffective exercises, it is first necessary to understand how the muscles work.

To lift a heavy object from a table, the proper muscles must first tense to the point that their strength equals that of the object. Only then can they shorten and move in order to lift the weight. The first part of this activity, the mere tensing, is called the isometric function of muscle activity; it consists exclusively in collecting strength. The lifting part of this activity is called isotonic muscle activity; it is the phase of the muscle-shortening that makes movement possible.

Our daily movements and activities consist mostly of these two kinds of exertion in various combinations. The skeletal muscles are built differently, depending on whether they function primarily as support or for movement. Depending on their tasks, muscles that function mostly statically fan out broadly, are flat, and have short fibers, while the muscles used for movement have long fibers to help carry out movements over several joints.

79

The basic principle of exercises to stimulate metabolism should not ignore the biological function of various muscles. The exercises should train the muscles' specific functions—i.e., the support muscles should be trained for strength and movement muscles trained through movement.

Isometric tension, which is held for six or more seconds, results in an intra-muscular pressure that is greater than the capillary pressure. This causes a decreased blood supply to the particular muscle. Since the muscle can no longer meet the heightened energy need by an increased blood supply, it must draw instead on the inner muscular reserve. This results in quickened combustion processes and in the accumulation of metabolic waste. In addition, any strong muscle tension leads to holding the breath in, because the use of the abdominal pressure reflexively stops the breathing movement. This further diminishes circulation to a muscle used for support. A muscle trained in this fashion quickly experiences a shortage of oxygen and tires quickly.

*Constant muscle tension results in oxygen shortage*

A true recovery effect for a muscle can only occur through frequent alternation between tension and release, allowing it sufficient time to regenerate. Exercises that stimulate breathing and circulation are also beneficial, for they assure a supply of oxygen to the muscle.

# Withstanding Cold

Conditioning has already been discussed on page 51 in connection with sciatica. In my practice I see many patients who complain of rheumatic problems. They spoil themselves with overheated apartments, lack of fresh air, and excessively warm clothing. As a result, they make themselves very sensitive to cold. Therefore, an additional word should be said on this subject, because only systematic conditioning really helps.

*Condition oneself against cold or continue to freeze?*

A characteristic sign of such patients having rheumatic complaints is that they freeze, with every draft, suffer neck pain from every slightly opened window, and suffer from cold painful knees despite wool socks or underwear. In the winter they get a succession of colds and because of their sensitivity are very susceptible to any form of flu, cold virus, and bronchitis. All these manifestations of colds are accompanied by diffuse pain in the arms and legs, muscles and joints.

How is conditioning achieved and what exactly should be done?

At the outset, let me say that conditioning cannot be achieved immediately; it is a long process. But if the effort is not abandoned with the first lapse into catching a cold, it is usually possible to break the vicious circle of susceptibility.

# Why People Feel the Cold Keenly

*Improper clothing*

Many things can cause a person to feel very cold. Some important reasons may be excessively low blood pressure or insufficient metabolism. Many young women feel the cold because of improper diets in an effort to get or stay thin. Such diets are often deficient in the calorie content needed to provide warmth from within. Sometimes improper clothing can also be at fault, especially synthetics whose fiber structure does not form an insulating layer of air and cannot hold warmth. This causes slight perspiration and results in constant cold due to evaporation. It typically results in cold feet or in a feeling of cold in the kidney area. A prerequisite to being warm is therefore to wear clothing that is porous rather than heavy. It should be made of natural fibers such as wool or cotton. There must also be adequate muscle metabolism to provide internal warmth, because the metabolism functions as a warming agent. Proper functioning of blood pressure is also important for warmth.

# The Ability to Adjust to Different Temperatures

Blood pressure can be raised in the morning by Kneipp's method of cold water treatment. It is of primary importance that each arm and leg be passed under a solid sheet of water. To do so, remove the shower head and train the hose directly over the surface of the body. Begin the treatment on the right leg, direct the water spray up along the back side of the leg up to the hollow of the knee, then to the groin or to the buttocks. The left leg is then similarly treated, then the right and left arm, finally the torso. Briefly washing with cold water also suffices. Movement also increases blood pressure—jumping, walking quickly, walking up the stairs rapidly instead of taking the elevator, walking a child to school, shopping by bicycle instead of by car. Instead of telephoning a co-worker in the office, go and visit him. All these activities provide warmth and activate metabolism. A vigorous exercise program is also warming, especially if done with the window open.

*Measures to promote body warmth*

Brush massage used in connection with a cold shower or an alternating cold-hot shower is effective in stimulating circulation, especially if done with the windows open. Once again, start with the right leg and brush in a circular motion from the bottom up, until you feel altogether warm from the inside.

Walking barefoot in a house that has carpets, parquet flooring and central heating and is usually warm, one will discover that the feet may be surprisingly warmer than with synthetic sox and shoes. If there is a possibility of stepping barefoot on dew-covered grass in the morning, this, too, will keep the feet warm for a good part of the day.

*Acclimatization to temperature can be learned*

Our evenly heated apartments no longer necessitate our circulation to acquire the ability to adjust to different temperatures. We must consciously do so by taking alternating hot and cold showers. Taking a short cold shower during the summer, and opening up the windows in seasons of transition or even in winter are recommended. Wearing lighter clothing in the house, going barefoot, using every opportunity even on cold days to move about outdoors for a short time are all effective measures.

The sauna is also a useful conditioning method, because it requires the circulation to be capable of adjusting. Keep in mind that high temperature differences require a robust circulation. Persons with low blood pressure (hypotension) as well as those with high blood pressure (hypertension) must be cautious. Where there is hypotension, a "bogging down" of too much blood in the skin can cause a lack of blood in the brain, resulting in dizziness and fainting. Where there is hypertension, an increase in pressure can result from an increase in the total blood supply.

# 6. The Extent to Which Muscles Can Be Trained

## The Problem of the Anonymous Exerciser

*Goal of physical training*

Training does not offer opportunities for the relaxing movement characteristic of sport and play activity. Training always has a goal and a reason. It focuses on certain muscle groups or organs for a particular purpose. For example, jumping requires the training of one particular muscle while the limbs need training for swimming. A good physical condition is based on good circulation and breathing.

It is difficult to design a training program without knowing the person's specific situation. It is necessary to know their physical difficulties, deficiencies, endurance, and the condition of their circulatory system. It is necessary to know when the trainee holds his breath due to exertion, when his face gets flushed, and whether he has a fat abdomen, varicose veins, or high blood pressure. It is impossible to observe him during his exercise periods and, most importantly, there is no opportunity to tell him when he is exercising incorrectly. I plan and institute programs for my patients, I can correct them, give them tips and inspiration, and show them how to continue the exercises on their own.

*. . . if your heart functions properly*

Even a doctor who writes a book on heart-circulation training is making information available to the general public with which he has no contact. Since he does not know his audience, he may cautiously add, ". . . if your heart is in good order; otherwise consult your physician." Many people do not know that the vessels around the heart have already become constricted and think it is normal for rapid walking to cause a fast pulse, shortness of breath, and heavy perspiration. They assume that they are utterly healthy and begin to train in order to get rid of these manifestations of fatigue. Actually most training is geared toward healthy, fit, slim, and agile persons and gives no consideration either to pathological changes that may already be present or to the aging process. Even if I often recommend swimming because it is excellent therapeutic movement, I must promptly modify the suggestion for many patients by adding, "Above all, swim on your back." The reason for doing so is that the strongly bent position of the head into the neck necessary for the breast stroke used by many older persons is detrimental to neck muscles already having a tendency toward cramping. The least harmful exercises are swimming, walking, a short run, and bicycle riding. These sports also have the advantage of being outdoor activities. They therefore stimulate breathing to a healthful, reasonable extent. Real training programs should be discussed and tested with a therapist. They should be geared to

*Valuable*
*training*
*disciplines*

the person doing them, to his needs and ability. They should be subject to being corrected at least once, otherwise they can do more harm than good.

Training through the aid of isometric exercises offers the advantage of strengthening a particular muscle, because these exercises increase the number and strength of the separate muscle fibers and aid in increasing the size of the muscle.

As a result of endurance training, however, the number of capillaries and oxygen supply in the given muscle increase. Since breathing is intensified, the lungs take in more oxygen, and the quantity of blood pumped by each beat of the heart is increased. Such endurance training can slowly be increased, but eventually reaches a limit beyond which nothing more can be achieved. This limit is naturally different for each individual.

*Do you know*
*the limit of*
*your ability?*

Many people, however, do not know their limitations and for this reason should first consult a physician familiar with their physical condition before starting a training program.

In general, the extent to which training can be successfully undertaken diminishes with increasing age. This diminution of physical efficiency can, however, within limits be postponed by a training program carefully tailored to the specific physiological capacity of the individual.

84

# The Proper Time for Training

A basic rule in every training program is regularity. Improvements achieved in the musculature and in the area of heart-circulation are quickly lost if the program is interrupted. The regularity of exercising is usually the weakest link in a chain of good intentions.

If you want a training program and have the time, tenacity, and are in condition to start it, schedule it for the time of day when you are at optimal physical capacity, which varies greatly in the course of the day. It peaks in the morning, drops considerably by noon, and increases in the late afternoon, although it never regains the level of the morning. For this reason, it would be senseless to use a noon break for exercising.

It is important to keep in mind, too, that psychological stress places a strain on the back, so in setting up an exercise program some consideration should be given to pleasure and gregariousness. A training program merely oriented toward sport and accomplishment will not succeed in bringing about relaxation and producing relief from back complaints. A feeling of vitality may sooner come from taking a hike with the family, a friend, and perhaps even with a mature son for whom you formerly never had time. Such relaxing activity offers opportunities for peaceful discussions, and the pleasures of enjoying company, movement, scenery, and fresh air all combine to increase vitality.

*Benefits of non-competitive activity*

# The Obsession with Fitness

Too many people—well meaning but misguided—try to correct years of neglect with one vigorous blow of exercise, with a sudden shape-up program. The obsession with fitness, which includes visits to health clubs even when it is not indicated therapeutically, is nourished by our wish to avoid growing old. Unfortunately it takes an increasingly heavy toll, as persons out of shape physically tear tendons, compress spines, and place demands on their circulation that result in acute lack of oxygen. Their running and jogging lead fairly directly to heart attacks. Even cross-country skiing, certainly a sport that can be beneficial and relaxing, often results in Loipen stress from

*Danger from the strain of cross-country skiing*

attempting to cover too great distances in too short a period of time. These remarks are merely another reminder that the prerequisite of a training program is patience for the slow process of building up endurance.

# 7. Self-Help Program for Back Pain

## The Prevention Is Easier Than the Cure

*Gymnastics without danger*

Preventive gymnastics is an attempt to activate the spinal column to make the ligaments and joints flexible, the chest cavity elastic, and to loosen up the musculature. A yoga course or a gymnastics class conducted by a community center or sports club offers the advantage of supervised exercise and the stimulation of group contact. Preventive gymnastics includes several basic exercises that are helpful and effective, and which can be practiced by anyone without risk or danger. However, if there is already some form of cervical or lumbar vertebral problem present, any exercise program, even a preventive program, should be preceded by medical physiotherapy. In such instances, training in specific exercises directed toward those particular complaints should be given before the person attempts to practice them alone.

*Test exercises by Professor Kraus*

To test your own muscular ability, I would like to present a group of exercises known as the Kraus-Weber Tests. Developed many years ago in the United States by Professor Hans Kraus, these tests, although not a gauge of flexibility (which is so important for the spinal column), test the strength and functioning of a muscle.

1. To test the groin, lie flat on the floor on your back with legs extended. Fold the hands under the head and hold the legs out

straight about 10 inches above the floor for 10 seconds.
2. Test the hip and stomach muscles by sitting up from a lying position while keeping the legs straight and hands folded behind the head.
3. The stomach muscles alone are tested by getting up from a reclining position with the knees bent, hands crossed behind the neck.
4. Test the back muscles by lying on the stomach and lifting the torso (put a hard pillow or bolster under yourself). Hold for 10 seconds. For this exercise, too, the hands are folded behind the neck.
5. The muscles of the lower back and buttocks are tested by lifting the legs from the same starting position as exercise 4.
6. Test the ability of the back leg muscles to stretch by standing straight and touching the floor with the fingertips without bending the knees.

With the exception of the first exercise, you need a partner to either hold down your feet or the small of the back (while lying on your stomach or back). This test does not deal with flexibility of the spinal column, CVC syndrome, a hip joint arthrosis, nor a Scheuermann round back. It is intended solely as a means of determining the strength of muscles in the torso.

# Setting up the Exercise Program

Most books offer several gymnastic exercises for the same condition or for a specific muscle group. It is recommended that you first read them through, then try one or two exercises you have understood to see if it serves your particular need. Consider also what really may be helpful.

Are you looking for a possibility of stretching your neck while sitting at a desk? An exercise for limbering up the lumbar vertebral column? An exercise to stimulate circulation after a long car ride, or an exercise for strengthening the abdominal muscles because you spend too much time sitting? Test and select exercises that may best serve specific needs, so that when the occasion arises you will know how to stretch the right spot effectively.

*Exercise slowly at first*

It is best to practice different movements slowly in the

beginning for the purpose of understanding, feeling, and controlling them, and by doing so to learn what is happening during an exercise and where. The tempo of an exercise should be increased only after it has become familiar. In this way one learns where and why problems arise with certain exercises, while others seem to feel right.

It is important to do the exercises correctly and to guard against creating difficulties by allowing errors to creep in.

Proceed slowly. It is far more effective to do a few exercises well than to do many exercises incorrectly.

*It is impor-*
*tant to have*
*a feeling for*
*your body*

Those persons who most need gymnastics often have astonishingly little feeling for their bodies and little or no feeling at all for the small of the back. Thus a simple bending and straightening motion of the pelvis is perceived as a difficulty. In a seated position, they move the torso only slightly back and forth without actually moving anything in the small of the back. At the beginning of an exercise intended to develop control in the lumbar vertebral column, place both hands under the small of the back on the pelvis, move slowly back and forth in order to feel what, if anything at all, moves in this area.

Every exercise should have a definite beginning and should have a well worked-out ending. After energetically doing limbering-up exercises, it is especially important for the body to regain a certain amount of tension. The closing accent of an exercise should promote the satisfying feeling of really having accomplished something.

*Correct*
*choice of*
*exercises*

In selecting exercises, take into consideration the various possible starting positions. Whenever possible, choose exercises that use the same starting position. In other words, choose those that start either from a sitting, standing, or lying position in order to avoid too much commotion in executing them. A smooth exercise program is satisfying, while an uneven one causes listlessness.

In the beginning, choose exercises for which you have sufficient strength and flexibility and which you can do well. Unsuccessful beginnings frequently lead to abandoning all good intentions toward taking exercises. Don't be afraid either of repeating an exercise. A program may be short and even relatively one-sided, but should be done as regularly as possible.

Remember that you are not always equally fit and productive and that everyone, by no means only women, is subject to fluctuations. The weather, an approaching cold, or emotional

*Amount of exercise determined by fitness and mood on a given day*

upsets can all strongly affect physical capacity. In choosing the exercises and the duration of the exercise session, take your mood at the time into consideration. Signs of overexertion are shortness of breath, a rapid pulse that does not return to normal within five minutes, a feeling of weakness and lassitude. This should not, however, be confused with a feeling of justifiable physical fatigue. In itself, perspiring is not harmful, but it should not be immoderate. A tendency to perspire is related to fluid intake, of course. It also varies with the individual—some persons are more inclined to perspire than others—and with temperature changes.

From all that has been stated thus far, it clearly emerges that there is much overlapping within separate groups of back complaints. Certain symptoms such as myogelosis are frequently manifested, and many syndromes mesh without having any specific delineations. Suggestions for therapy will therefore include duplications. Many of the exercises are suitable for back pain in general, regardless of its genesis. Similarly, various occupations and groups of occupations are disposed toward several complexes of symptoms—for example, toward both LVC and CVC syndromes. An enumeration of various occupations and their susceptibility to certain back changes must necessarily always be incomplete. Such a list can at best only provide general characteristics and indicators concerning the category of complaint into which the individual may fit.

# Preventive Measures for Myogelosis

The syndrome was described in detail on page 27.

*Almost everyone has muscle hardenings*

**Appearance.** Knotty hardening of the muscles, chiefly in the neck and shoulder musculature or in the muscles between the shoulder blades and the spinal column; muscle hardening like cords in the area of the small of the back.

**Complaints.** Piercing pain, sometimes a burning sensation in the affected muscle parts, especially after prolonged sitting, radiating pain to the head and arms, a tendency for the hands to fall asleep at night.

### Frequently affected occupations

1. Sedentary occupations: people who work at desks—as, for example, students and lawyers, secretaries; men and women who work at machines; workers on assembly lines; technical draftsmen; watchmakers, jewelers, etc.
2. Occupations that combine sitting, driving and a high degree of concentration such as taxi drivers, pilots, salesmen, long distance drivers, private chauffeurs, crane operators, tractor drivers, etc.
3. Persons in general stress situations: housewives who have children and a job, persons with occupational-financial-family problems, persons who have insomnia, or vegetative dystonia.

### A doctor's therapeutic measures

*Seek treatment promptly*

Diagnose and explain the existing pain. Treatment includes medication, radiotherapy, electrotherapy.

### Physiotherapeutic measures

Massages, underwater massage, heat applications, stretching and relaxation exercises, gymnastics to improve circulation.

### Preventive aids

1. Alternating hot and cold showers directed toward the affected muscles.
2. Brush massage to stimulate circulation of affected muscles.
3. Hand massage (self-massage).
4. Learning to relax by studying autogenic training.
5. Gymnastics.

*This is how it is done*

*Atlernating hot and cold showers.* Always begin with warm water and end with a cold phase. There should be the greatest possible contrast between hot and cold temperatures. The change from hot to cold should be rapid and is best accomplished by having a container of cold water ready from which you can dip to pour over yourself. A hot shower lasting

91

about 2 minutes should be followed by a short cold phase. Total direction about 10 minutes. Result: lively feeling of warmth throughout.

*Brush massage.* Using a long-handled massage brush or a coarse sponge, vigorously brush the affected musculature. It is preferable to have a partner work on your back from the lower part up—i.e., starting from the small of the back and the rear of the pelvis. Circular motions should be used.

*Hand massage (self-massage).* Without too much difficulty you can work on your own neck muscles and knead them. The problem in doing so is to relax one part of your body while the other is working. This can be done successfully by lying on your side and supporting the upper arm at the waist, letting it fall loosely forward with the shoulder. It can also be done sitting if you place your arm on the back rest of a chair or couch, a position that will relax the neck muscles on that side of the body. Reaching over with the other hand, you can then grasp and knead the muscles. It is possible to rapidly acquire a feeling for the main source of pain. Touch the muscle strand, press it vigorously between the thumb and other fingers and then massage it. Don't be shy about grasping it; even pull the muscle away from its underlying tissue and rotate one or two fingers over particularly hardened portions. Do this with as strong a grip as possible. You will rapidly acquire a sense for how much pressure to use.

*Relaxation can be learned*

*Autogenic training.* No one should attempt to learn this method of relaxation by themselves from books. Those persons most in need of relaxation have great difficulties in learning it. They often quickly reach a dead end, causing them to doubt the method and abandon any further efforts. If they had sought instruction either from a medical source or from some school, they could have been helped to overcome their difficulty and would not have lost a valuable possibility of physical and mental regeneration.

*Gymnastics.* Before getting out of bed:
• Lie on your back, fold hands under your neck so the area between neck and head rests between the cushions of the thumbs. Use the hands for pulling the head forward and upward, let the tension work for about 3 seconds, then lay the head back against the pressure of the hands, press firmly on the support for

*Getting up begins while still in bed*

3 seconds, release, and consciously relax again. Repeat two or three times.

• Lie on your back, rest arms loosely at the sides of your body. Push arms down tightly against the bed so the entire shoulder and shoulder blade musculature tenses. Hold tension for 3 seconds, then release it completely, breathe deeply in order to enjoy the relaxation, then begin again. Repeat 3 times.

• Sit on the edge of the bed, lift arms and stretch vigorously. With arms up, alternately bend the torso slightly to each side, energetically stretching up the outside arm into the direction of the bend. Coordinate each stretching motion with a deep breath. Do the exercise twice slowly on each side.

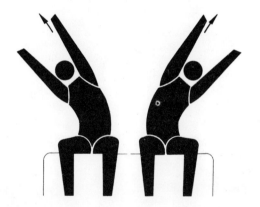

*Morning exercises on the edge of the bed*

• Sit on the edge of the bed, round the back as much as possible, making certain to include the cervical vertebral column; with the head bent down, stretch the arms forward until tension is felt between the shoulder blades. Then stretch the back and pull the shoulder blades back together as far as possible. Repeat 3 times.

• Stand and loosely move the shoulders in a circle with arms hanging down. Do this five times in each direction.

• Alternately raise the right and left shoulders in rapid succession, simultaneously letting the upper body roll forward slightly until the arms alternately almost touch the floor. Straighten up slowly. Do this exercise energetically without tensing. Repeat twice.

• In a standing position, fold hands over the head and stretch arms up as if one arm wanted to pull the other out of the body. Maintain the tension and slowly roll the torso toward until the main tension and the apex of the curve are between the shoulder blades. Slowly straighten up; repeat three times.

• Begin in the same way as the last exercise. After attaining optimal tension with the spinal column bent, unclasp the hands, let the torso hand down limply and let the arms dangle like pendulums. Then slowly raise the torso, simultaneously turning it so energetically to each side that the loosely hanging arms are included in the movement. The arms virtually swing out behind the torso. When fully stretched, lift arms sideways until perpendicular, then slowly, while feeling they are being stretched into the fingertips, bring them down to the side.

Keep in mind that all stretching exercises require time and that they should be done slowly.

*Restore body tension at the end*
Vigorous exercises should always end with a slightly accentuated tension in order to regain total body tension.

Remember, too, the necessity of a pleasing ending.

**Relaxation for people who work at desks**

• Rest both elbows on top of the desk and put the forehead in the hands. Press elbows so firmly on the desk that the muscles between the shoulder blades tense. Maintain the tension for three counts, and release. Loosely moving the shoulders in a circle, repeat as needed.

*Exercise for people who work at desks*

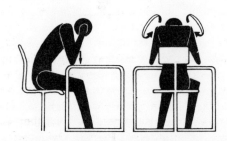

• Place underarms parallel to body on desk and push out and round the spinal column, then pull it back in. If this movement is done in an unforced and flowing manner, it carries over to the cervical vertebrae column and head, which loosely participate in the movement.

• Fold the arms loosely, extend them horizontally from the body and move them to the right and to the left so the shoulder blades glide back and forth. Do this several times to each side.

• Stretch the back and roll the head slowly from one side across the front to the other and back.

• Lean the head to the side so the ear almost touches the shoulder. Reach with one hand over the head to the other ear so the weight of the hand contributes to the stretching of the side throat muscles. While applying a counterforce with the hand, raise the head again after two or three seconds. Do the same on the other side.

• Stretch the torso and turn the head as far as possible to the right, hold the tension briefly, then in a similar manner turn energetically to the left, tense briefly and release. Repeat three times on each side.

*Exercise for people who work at desks*

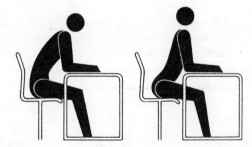

• Place the arms on top of the desk. Pull the head as far as possible into the shoulders, then push it up again as far as possible. To strengthen the stretching ability of the throat muscles, pull chin down toward throat. Repeat several thimes.

• Loosely raise shoulders, then let them drop back down. Repeat several times. Practice this exercise quickly and springily.

95

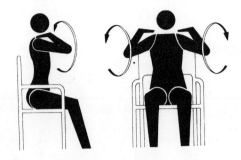

• Place hands on shoulders with the elbows at right angles to the body. Make large circular motions with the elbows. Practice both toward the front and back.

• Hold yourself on the front edge of a chair and press the back against the pulling tension of the arms as far as possible. The back should be rounded. Then stretch the back again until the shoulder blades almost touch, maintaining the pull in the arms. Change the direction several times, then limber up the shoulders again by a slight circling motion.

**Relaxation exercises for car drivers**

*Exercises for drivers*

• Making large swinging motions with the torso is beneficial after long hours of driving. Raise the arms. Let the torso swing down vigorously, then raise it again. Keep the knees flexible so that they, too, are involved in the movements of the torso.

• Stand with legs spread apart and turn the torso so vigorously from side to side that the arms are flung out from the body. The movement is initiated by the pelvis.

• Stand with legs spread apart, raise arms and alternately touch fingertip to foot on opposite side. Do this vigorously, repeat several times.

96

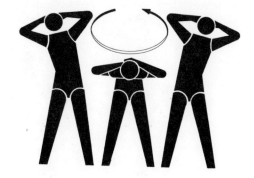

• Stand with legs spread apart, hands folded behind the neck, and loosely incline upper body to the side down toward the front, and then turn toward other side. Take care that the upper body stays to the front and does not turn during the motions toward the side. Stand up straight again, stretch arms, and bring them down to the sides.

*Keep the pulse in mind and don't overexert*

• To improve circulation, run in place for a brief period of time. Do so until breathing is stimulated, but not to the point of feeling shortness of breath. The pulse should be back to normal within 5 minutes.

• The same effect can be achieved by standing with legs together and hopping lightly on one spot. Alternately hop like a jumping jack by hopping with legs spread apart and hands clasped over the head. The arms should remain taut while doing the exercise.

• Stand with legs slightly spread apart. Push the small of the back out, then pull it in toward the hollow of the back. If the pelvis is shifted slightly to the side, the pelvis will rotate loosely.

97

• To loosen up the small of the back, walk forward with arms held at an angle. With each step, pull the other knee so high that, with the help of a slight turn and bend of the torso, the knee and elbow of opposite sides almost touch.

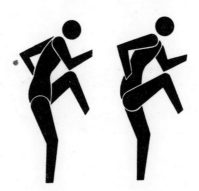

*Exercises for drivers*

• Crank each arm briefly like a windmill. After doing this with each arm, bring both arms up vertically, alternately stretch out the fingers energetically and make a fist. Bring arms down to side again.

**General relaxation exercises**

*Different ways of relieving muscle tension*

Anyone who has studied autogenic training learns how to relax for short periods in any situation. But even persons who have not mastered autogenic methods will always find opportunities to relax that are refreshing and helpful. Sometimes it can be done by breathing, at other times by energetically tensing the muscles.

*Self-observation is relaxing*

• Pull your legs up and sit crosslegged on a chair. Support the underarms on the thighs, letting the hands fall between the knees and letting the head hang down limply. Close your eyes and try to observe your breathing motions, merely following their up and down motions without exerting any influence on the breathing. This position is so relaxing that it is almost possible to doze off. It is not surprising that it was used in former times by coach drivers for relaxing while filling periods of waiting, and that is why it is called the "coachman's position." (Open the waistband if necessary to be able to breathe deeply.)

• The same relaxation can be achieved while lying down merely by observing the in-and-out breathing rhythm of the abdominal wall. Put a pillow under the hollow of the knees or preferably under the whole lower leg. Keep arms slightly bent beside the body.

• Lie on the floor and rest the lower legs on the seat of a chair or sofa. Push yourself up from the floor so the body is stretched out and tensed, and supported only by the shoulders and lower legs. Hold this position for several seconds, then return to the relaxed starting position and breathe deeply and quietly. This can be repeated after a few minutes and should be followed by a period of relaxation and deep breathing.

*Relaxation and breathing exercise*

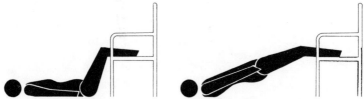

• Lie down on the back. Pull the knees up close to the abdomen and wrap the arms around them so the head almost touches the knees. Hold this position for several seconds, then stretch out completely, relax. Breathe quietly.

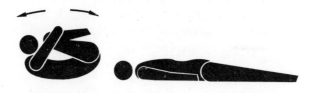

*Relaxation and breathing exercise*

• Making a big turn with the torso is also relaxing and is an effective way of limbering up. Start by keeping knees flexible while raising the arms. Bend the torso and let it dangle down like a pendulum. Then straighten the knees, tense the upper body and straighten up like a folding pocket knife in order to regain total tension. Lower the arms to the side.

99

# Measures for LVC Syndrome and Disc Damage

The syndrome was described in detail on page 39.

**Appearance.** Frequently a hollow back with very braced back extensor muscles that are visible and look like thick ropes next to the spinal column. Sometimes accompanied by swelling of the tissue across the small of the back.

*One of the most frequent syndromes*

**Complaints.** Dull pain in the small of the back, especially across the sacrum and at the transition from the sacrum to the lumbar vertebrae. Radiating pains into the leg (sciatic irritation). Sometimes piercing pain while turning or bending. Pain in the small of the back upon awakening in the morning, which disappears by moving about slowly.

### Frequently affected occupations

All sitting occupations if the seating is poor or the work surfaces too low, and occupations that combine driving and sitting—i.e., secretaries, students, scholars, bookkeepers, taxi drivers, long distance drivers, school children whose desks are too small.

All standing occupations that do not allow enough change of body position—i.e., salespersons, cashiers, workers on assembly lines and many others.

Occupations involving lifting and carrying—such as furniture movers, mailmen, beer truck drivers, stockroom workers, factory workers, construction workers, farmers, and others.

Unsuitable sports: tennis, golf, and soccer.

### Therapeutic measures by a doctor

*Importance of diagnosis*

Providing an accurate diagnosis and making a clear distinction between back problems and gynecological or urological syndromes. Use of medication for severe pain. If neurological symptoms such as numbness or muscular weakness are present, recommendation of chiropractic or surgical treatment. Electrotherapy, radiotherapy.

**Physiotherapeutic measures**

Warmth, traction (stretching by pulling) by use of apparatus (traction, tilted board), underwater massage, massage of fibrous tissue, stretching and mobilization exercises, gymnastics.


**Preventive self-help**

1. Warmth by use of a heating pad.
2. Hot showers, especially for the small of the back area.
3. Warm baths with gentle attempts at mobilization.
4. Gymnastics.

Regarding 1. Put a heating pad or warm blanket under the small of the back and prop up the legs so that the hip and knee joints are bent at right angles and the small of the back sags. For this purpose, loose chair seats can be stacked up, or a stool can be stacked with pillows and blankets, or the seat of a chair can be used for propping up the lower legs while lying on the floor. The head can be supported by a flat pillow.

*Unburdening brings relief*

Regarding 2. A hot shower aimed at the painful area in the small of the back in the morning and also at night before retiring is an effective aid in releasing tension.

Regarding 3. While in a warm bath, draw up the legs and push the small of the back down, then release; repeat several times.
    With the legs similarly bent and drawn up, push one knee so far forward that the pelvis participates in the movement while the thighs remain parallel and close together.
    Let the bent legs fall first to one side, then to the other.

Regarding 4. *Gymnastics* before getting out of bed.
• Lie sprawled out on your back, and stretch vigorously. Bring one leg up to the abdomen, wrap the arms around it and pull it tightly toward the body, then stretch it out again. Repeat with the other leg.
• Bring both legs to the abdomen, wrap the arms around them and, guided by the breathing rhythm, pull them close and release—i.e., while inhaling, pull them in; while exhaling, release them.

101

• Bend your knees and let them rest loosely against the body. Use your hands to move the bent legs back and forth in a circular motion. The movement should feel pleasant, especially in the small of the back. Circle in both directions, then slowly straighten legs again.

• Rest the arms on the edge of the bathtub, stretch and round out the small of the back, then pull it in toward the slight lordosis. Repeat several times.

*Exercises for the lumbar spinal column:*

• Lie down on the back, bend legs at the knees and hips, and vigorously push the small of the back down to the floor several times. Then raise the buttocks from the floor, briefly hold the position, and lower again. Then resume original position. As a variation of the same exercise, after raising the buttocks, push the pelvis slightly to the side and rest it there. Then bring the buttocks over to the other side in an arch so that each movement now describes a large half-circle. In ending the exercise, return to the center.

*Get to know the right pelvic position*

• Extend the legs, and alternately stretch them so far out from the body that the pelvis also moves.

• Stand on all fours, arch the back like a cat, then push the small of the back in the opposite direction so it hangs down somewhat. Practice this movement slowly, repeating it several times and permitting the cervical vertebral column and head to participate in the movement.

• If you have mastered the previous exercise, while arching your back, shift the weight to the rear so that you are almost sitting on your heels. Then push the torso flatly forward between the arms, which are now bent, meantime lifting your head. Then start over again by arching your back.

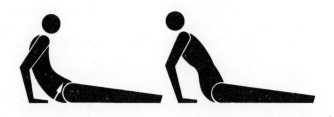

*Exercises for pelvic flexibility*

102

• Sit with the legs extended. Raise the torso by placing the hands behind the body for support so the small of the back is limply curved outward. Slowly pull the pelvis forward until the back is as straight as possible, then let it become limp again. Repeat several times.

• While sitting on your heels or in a cross-legged position, the lumbar vertebral column provides most of the support. Assume either position, and keep the shoulder girdle rigid by holding a stick or tautly-held towel above your head. (When sitting on the heels, the back of the foot, or the instep, is flat on the floor.) With the arms still raised, incline the torso to one side, bending and twisting around to the other side and back, describing a half-circle. Straighten up the torso and return to the frontal position. Repeat several times.

• Stand with legs apart, arms raised, incline the torso loosely to one side so one arm hangs down and the other rests lightly on the head. Vigorously turn to the other side. Keep in mind that when facing forward that you should be fully stretched before letting the torso fall over to the other side.

• Same position as the previous exercise, but now instead of stretching between changing sides, bend the torso sharply and swing it over to the other side. Then stand up straight, facing forward before continuing to other side. Repeat several times to each side. Bring legs together and slowly straighten up.

• Stand with legs spread apart, arms raised. Alternately touch fingertip to opposite foot. Practice energetically; repeat several times.

• The whole back can be limbered up by raising the arms, bending the torso forward, and then letting the arms and head dangle loosely while keeping the knees flexible and springy. While in this position, let the arms and head swing back and forth before tensing, standing up straight, and stretching all the way to the fingertips.

*Taking the pressure off the spinal column*

*To release tension after sitting a long time*

• Hold yourself on the edge of a chair and let the pelvis hang loosely toward the back, then pull it back to the front to form a slight hollow in the back. Gradually include a side movement of the pelvis until it makes a circular motion. Repeat several times loosely in both directions.

• Using your arms, briefly lift yourself from the seat of the chair so the spinal column is temporarily relieved of pressure.

103

• Let the torso hang down between your legs, then slowly raise and stretch it upward.
• Alternately pull the right and left knees up to your nose. You may use your hands to help.
• Stretch out completely on the chair for a brief period of time. Stretch the hip joints and knees. Also stretch the arms up high and stretch the head up from the neck so the back tenses like an arch, then release.

# Measures for a Round Back

*A round back can still be corrected during childhood*

The syndrome was described in detail on page 53.

**Appearance.** Clearly visible bending of the thoracic spinal column. The condition can often be corrected in children, but among adults it is permanent because the individual vertebral bodies have become deformed, assumed a wedge shape, and have so adjusted to the curvature that the spinal column can no longer straighten out even when lying on the stomach. The condition is especially pronounced in Scheurmann's disease, which was described on page 55, and in instances of general weakness of the tissues and tendons.

**Complaints.** Very tense musculature, especially between the shoulder blades; back pain on overexertion, as in long sitting or standing; back tires rapidly; occasional sensitivity of some vertebrae to pressure; frequent pain in the small of the back due to compensatory lordosis; great tautness of the extensor muscles in the area of the small of the back.

**Occupations conducive to syndrome**

In general, all leptosomatic persons who are thin, who grew very tall rapidly, frequently characterized by weak ligaments, limbs, and a somewhat distinct musculature. Males are usually affected.

Tall persons who sit while working—office workers, researchers, and students, including persons whose work requires standing, such as salespersons, waiters, etc.

Young workers and apprentices who at an early age had to lift and carry heavy objects.

104

### Therapeutic measures undertaken by a doctor

An accurate diagnosis, especially of young males, is vital for early detection of Scheuermann's disease before bone breaks and deformation of the vertebrae occur *(see p. 56)*. For advanced cases, a cast worn while sleeping may be necessary. Medication to promote and support bone and tissue development is usually indicated.

### Physiotherapeutic measures

*Stretching, mobilizing, strength- ening*

Stretching of the tissues, especially those of the front armpit, which is always braced and shortened, mobilization of the spinal column to the extent still possible, strengthening of the back musculature through well-chosen orthopedic exercises, instruction in good posture, massages.

### Preventive self-help

1. Well-chosen gymnastics.
2. Sports for children: swimming, rowing, "push-pull cars."
3. Sports for adults: rowing, surfing, gymnastics using such equipment as rings, horizontal bar, swimming.
    Stretching the front chest musculature is especially important for a round back, and in my view should be the beginning of every exercise program.

*Regarding 1. Stretching exercises.*
• Fold hands in back of the neck, lean into a half-opened door so that one elbow supports you on the door jam and the other elbow on the outer edge of the door. Lean into your arms; you must feel the pull in front of the armpits. Hold for at least 10 seconds, flex the knees occasionally. Repeat two to three times.
• Hang on a horizontal bar. Perhaps one can be installed in the door jam. A word of caution: most closet doors in contemporary buildings are not built sturdily enough to take the weight of an adult.
• Kneel down, sit on your heels, and push arms forward as far as possible on the floor. Lift your buttocks up so the arms slide somewhat further forward and the back stretches. By now, only

the lower legs, knees and hands are on the floor. Hold this stretching position for at least 10 seconds, then resume the position of sitting with the buttocks on the heels. Repeat two or three times.

*Exercises to strengthen the back muscles*
• Lie on your stomach on the floor, arms extended. Grasp two legs of a chair right under the seat with both hands. Lift the head and torso as far as possible from the floor. Hold a few seconds and lie down again. Breathe deeply. Make certain that the head remains approximately level with the torso. Avoid pulling the head too vigorously into the neck.

*Stretching the back is important*

• Lie on your stomach, stretch the right arm and left leg well away from the body, lift them just off the floor, hold for 3 seconds and bring them down again. Then practice the other diagonal. Repeat each side vigorously four to five times.
• For this exercise, you will need a partner or may use a piece of furniture to anchor your feet. Try to lift both arms simultaneously, hold briefly, then lower them. Guard against stretching the head too much into the neck in order to avoid cramping of the neck musculature.
• It is easier for heavier or older persons to do the previous exercise from an all-fours or crawling position. In this position, hip joints and knees form a right angle and so does the shoulder-arm connection. The arms are stretched, hands slightly turned in to avoid straining the elbows. Now lift right arm and left leg simultaneously until both are horizontal. Hold, put down and change sides—i.e., left arm with right leg. Repeat each side five times.

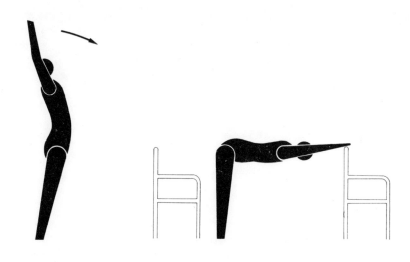

• Stand, legs spread apart, arms raised and stretched. Bend
down toward a chair until the arms rest on top of the back of the
chair. While doing so, stretch the thoracic part of the spine.
Move up and down a few times and continue stretching while
returning to upright position. Repeat a few times.
• Stand, hands folded behind neck. Bend torso slightly, until the
apex of the curve is just behind the shoulder blades. While
applying a counterforce with your hands, slowly resume upright
position. Pull elbows back to shoulder line. Repeat several
times.
• With arms outstretched, bend the upper body forward until
arms are horizontal. Hold briefly, then let arms fall down limply
and bob up and down a few times so the knees are also involved.
Tense again, and straighten up like an open pocket knife. Lower
arms to side.
• Pushups are often recommended for round backs. Pushups are
done by lying on the stomach, bracing against the floor with
outstretched arms, and pushing up the body while holding it stiff
like an inclined board. That is, the body is supported only by the
hands and feet. This exercise, however, requires a great deal of
strength and is really only suitable for males. For older and less
athletically trained persons, it is preferable to vary this exercise
in such a way that its effectiveness for the back is scarcely
diminished: lie on your stomach on the floor, place the legs on a
chair without arm rests or on an upholstered stool. By

*A pushup
that all can
do*

107

supporting the arms on the floor, it is possible to bend and stretch them slowly several times, causing the back to stretch in the area of the thoracic part of the spine. Done in this manner, it is as effective as the conventional, more strenuous pushup.

# Measures for CVC Syndrome

The syndrome was described in detail on page 59.

**Appearance.** Cartilage and bone changes in the area of the cervical vertebral column and the small cervical vertebral joints.

*CVC syndrome is a scourge*

**Complaints.** Painful muscle tensing, impaired movement in the throat and neck area, radiating headache, dizziness, migraine, shoulder-arm pain and shoulder-arm stiffness. Hands fall asleep at night.

**Occupations conducive to syndrome**

1. Occupations requiring a one-sided position of the body, such as dentists, cashiers, assembly line workers, sewing machine operators, farmers who while driving a tractor turn around to check on the machinery being pulled by the tractor.
2. Occupations that require working with raised arms so the head is pushed down into the neck—for example, assembly line workers in the automobile industry, computer workers, window washers, painters, etc.
3. Taxi drivers who sit too low. Seating that is too low forces the person to raise the chin, thereby pushing the head into the neck until the entire throat-neck area is cramped.

**Therapeutic measures undertaken by a doctor**

Clarification of the specific diagnosis, perhaps recommending chiropractic manipulation of a slightly slipped vertebral joint, medication in the event of dizziness and deficient circulation to the brain and, if needed, migraine therapy; radiotherapy; electrotherapy.

## Physiotherapeutic measures

*Avoid too
frequent use
of traction*

Traction—i.e., stretching by pulling of the cervical vertebrae. This can better be controlled manually than by an apparatus for applying traction (Glisson's sling). Special tensing and movement exercises, especially resistance exercises for the musculature of the cervical vertebral column. Careful mobilization movements or the cervical vertebral column, massages, warmth.

## Preventive self-help

1. Alternating hot and cold showers, particularly on the neck and shoulder musculature *(see page 82)*.
2. Brush massage *(see page 92)*.
3. Hand massage (self-massage) on the neck and throat muscles.
4. Gymnastics.

*Relief by
stretching*

*Regarding 4. Stretching exercises.* Since the complaints in a CVC syndrome frequently arise from fusion of discs and vertebrae in the throat area, stretching is a particularly effective source of relief.
• Bend over an easy chair or over the corner of the bed so that the head hangs down and the cervical vertebral column is curved with the head acting as weight. Stretching is increased by placing the folded hands on the head.
• Sit down and let the head hang down so the chin rests on the breastbone. This is effective in stretching the cervical vertebral column. The effect is strengthened by the weight of the folded hands on the head. Then push the head against the resistance of the weight of the hands and slowly straighten up again.
• Sit, fold the hands around the neck in such a way that the transition from the neck to the back of the head rests firmly in the balls of the hands. Forcefully press the head into the hands. The hands should not yield to the pressure but instead should pull the head up alternately to the right and to the left. After having stretched each side several times, the head should feel free and light.
• Let the head hang loosely forward. Use the shoulders to describe parallel small circles toward the front and back, almost as if making figure eights. Then roll the head languorously and slowly over the shoulders to the rear and return it to frontal

position. Repeat with other side before lifting the head again.
• Incline the head toward the side so the ear almost touches the shoulder. Reach with one hand over the head to the upper ear so the weight of the hand helps in stretching the lateral throat muscles. After 2 to 3 seconds, raise the head against the resistance of the hand. Repeat on other side.
• Stretch the torso and turn the head as far as possible to the right, maintain the tension briefly, then turn energetically toward the left, hold briefly, and release. Repeat three times on each side.
• Place arms on the surface of a table. Pull head in as far as possible between the shoulder blades, then push it up as far as possible out of the shoulders again. To increase the stretching of the throat muscles, also pull chin down to throat. Repeat several times.
• Pull the shoulders loosely up and down several times. Practice the up-and-down motion quickly.
• Place hands on shoulders, elbows at right angles to the body and describe large circles in the air. Practice several times toward front and back.

# Gymnastics for Postural Weakness

*How to prevent postural damage*

In general, all visible forms of postural deviations require orthopedic and physiotherapeutic treatment and cannot merely be treated by the use of exercise programs. But postural errors where the damage resulting from poor posture is hardly visible and cannot be felt can be treated by a muscle-strengthening regimen for the entire body. Above all, the abdominal muscles so important for posture should be exercised. What is meant by postural errors are actually marginal cases such as a slight lateral curvature of the spine that is visible only from the front when the torso is bent. Postural errors are the result of slight postural weakness, postural insecurity, and slight lack of muscle balance. For such cases, a strengthening program of gymnastics is the best form of prophylaxis.

**Exercises for abdominal muscles**

Like the back muscles, the abdominal muscles are arranged in

110

layers. Some of the fibers of these muscles run obliquely; those starting from the crest of the ilium run diagonally up, across, and down like the fingers of an open hand. The middle level supports the abdominal wall mainly with fibers that run diagonally. The deep level provides support with a broad, strong muscle that runs vertically from the breastbone and ribs to the pelvis. All these muscles functioning simultaneously are capable of extraordinary strength. But when they are weakened by inactivity or too much stretching as may occur from a large stomach, they even lack sufficient strength to provide abdominal muscular pressure for digestion. Constipation is in fact frequently caused by weakened abdominal muscles. Conversely, spastic constipation can be caused by heightened abdominal muscle tension, or cramping. In other words, the abdominal muscles are of critical importance to metabolism as well as to posture.

*Strengthening the abdominal muscles*

Since the fibers of the abdominal muscles run in several different directions, exercises for this area must be of several different kinds.

*Exercises for the straight abdominal muscles*
• Lie on your back, stretch arms forward, lift to a half sitting position, hold briefly and slowly lie back down.

*Abdominal muscle exercise on the floor*

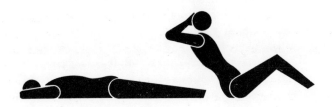

• Intensify the previous exercise by folding the hands behind the neck and bending the knees.
• Lie on your back, lift the legs until they are perpendicular to floor, then slowly lower them.
• In the same position, use your legs to simulate riding a bicycle vigorously. While doing so, gradually have the legs come closer to the floor but without touching it. Then raise legs until perpendicular. Slowly lower them while keeping them straight.
• Lift legs slightly from the floor and open and close several times in a scissor motion. To end the exercise, lift legs until

111

perpendicular and keep them straight while slowly bringing them down.

• Sit on the edge of a chair and hold the bottom of the back of a chair with both hands, bend the knees, pull them up, stretch them in front of you, hold briefly, and lower them.

• It is more difficult if one sits sideways so that the back of the chair is not in the way. To do so, fold the hands on the back of the neck, and while stretching the torso let it drop down toward the rear. Lean far enough back for the abdominal musculature to be able to support the weight of the body, but not so far that breathing is impeded. Slowly return to starting position.

• The previous exercise becomes even more effective by simultaneously doing the following: bend one leg, lift it, and then stretch it out high toward the front. Hold the position, then slowly lower. If you already have very strong abdominal muscles, lift both legs simultaneously, stretch them toward the front, hold, and then lower them.

• Squat on the floor with hands folded across the back of the neck. Lean the torso back and extend the legs diagonally forward into the air, hold briefly, then lower them.

*Exercises for the diagonal abdominal muscles*

• Lie on your back, legs slightly apart. Place one hand under the head and raise the head and shoulder of the same side until half sitting. Simultaneously lift opposite leg slightly, keeping both legs about a hand's width apart. Hold a few seconds and slowly lower them.

• Again lie on the back with legs slightly apart. Push the torso just enough to the side that it lies next to one leg. Raise yourself to a sitting position and move slightly up and down on that leg, then lie back down in the diagonal of the respective leg. The arms also participate in the forward movement.

• Sit down with legs straight ahead and slightly spread apart. Anchor them under a heavy piece of furniture (or have a partner hold them). With hands clasped behind the head and the torso stretched, lean back diagonally so far that the elbow of the same side almost touches the floor. Slowly straighten up again. Practice several times on each side.

• The following exercise is particularly effective for strengthening the muscles in the area of the stomach: lie down on your back, hands folded behind the neck, and knees bent. Lift yourself up, using only the head and shoulders, hold for a few seconds, and slowly lie back down. Repeat several times.

*Abdominal muscle exercise on a chair*

• An exercise particularly effective for the diagonal abdominal muscles: sit on the edge of a chair, and hold onto the bottom of the back of the chair. Bend the legs, stretch them diagonally and up, first to the right, then to the left, simultaneously leaning back with the upper body in the corresponding diagonal past the back of the chair.

Isometric exercises can perhaps be more effectively used for the abdominal muscles than for any other muscles. Often the abdominal muscles atrophy, causing both the number and thickness of the muscle fibers to decrease, so even their size needs to be improved.

If this is the case, pull the abdomen in as far as possible and hold the tension 5 to 6 seconds, then release. This exercise involves all the important abdominal muscle parts and, in order to be effective, should be repeated several times in succession every day.

*Exercises for the back muscles*

The back muscles are actually involved in all exercises requiring stretching of the back. This is true, regardless of the position— whether lying prone, squatting on the heels, sitting cross-legged, bending the torso while standing or walking to bring about a correction of posture. The fibrous portions of the back muscles are always involved in erecting and stretching the body.

*How to strengthen the back extensors*

• Lie on the stomach: alternately raise the forward-stretched arm and opposite leg, hold briefly, then lower. Before doing this exercise, it is important to stretch the arms. This is done by extending and stretching the arm and corresponding leg before lifting and tensing them.

• Lie on the stomach: lift both outstretched arms simultaneously, hold briefly, then lower. If you put a roll under the abdomen or have a partner hold down the small of the back, greater movement is possible than without assistance.

• In an all-fours position with a stretched back, lift the right leg and left arm to the height of the back—i.e., horizontally hold, then slowly lower. Practice other diagonal, repeating 3-5 times.

• Stand, with upper body held straight. Raise arms to a horizontal position, hold briefly. Then lower and swing them loosely while keeping the knees springy and responsive to the pendulum motion of the arms. Repeat, and end by lowering the arms.

• By stretching the head against the resistance of the hands folded on top of the head, the torso is stretched just as it would be by carrying something on the head or shoulders. This exercise can be done while standing or sitting and can be practiced at home by placing, for example, a package of laundry, a heavy book, or a briefcase on the head or by carrying a small child on the shoulders.

Carrying a weight on the head is an excellent diagnostic tool for persons lacking in feeling for their bodies and uncertain of the direction in which the torso should be stretched.

# 8. Preventive Measures for Persons without Back Problems

## Daily Exercises for Your Health

**An exercise program**

*Read carefully before trying out*

**1.** Lie on your back with arms next to the body and the legs straight. Lift legs until they are vertical, then vigorously move them as if riding a bicycle. While doing so, slowly lower the legs until they almost reach the floor, but avoid decreasing the intensity of movement, which now consists mainly in pulling in and stretching out the legs. Maintain pedaling motion while returning legs to vertical position. The feet are also involved in the pulling and stretching motions.
**2.** Keep the legs vertical and push them up still higher by providing support with your hands until the pelvis is also raised and you are actually resting on your shoulders.

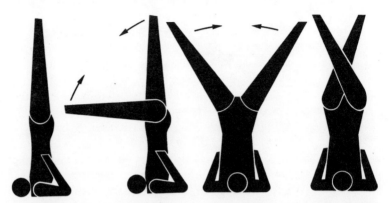

**3.** Holding the legs straight, lower one leg toward the front until it is at right angles with the other. Immediately return to original position and, alternating legs, exercise each side five times. Vary the motions by alternately closing and opening legs out to the side and by crossing the legs over each other.

**4.** In the same position of resting the weight of the body on the shoulders and providing some support with the hands, move the pelvis as far as possible to the right and left.

**5.** Slowly roll the torso back until it is completely flat again but keep legs vertical and together before lowering them slowly. Hold them just above the floor for 3 seconds before putting them down.

*Don't forget proper breathing*

**6.** Vigorously raise the torso to a sitting position and, without interrupting the movement, bend and kick the legs 3 times, then slowly lie back down again. Repeat 5 times.

**7.** Turn on your side, with one arm bent under the body and the head resting on it. Brace the other arm against the floor in front of the chest for support. Lift up the upper leg quickly and vigorously, making certain to stretch all the way to the toes. Repeat ten to fifteen times without interruption. Before returning to a rest position, hold the extended leg to the one on the floor for a few seconds, then lower it completely and practice the other side.

**8.** Roll on your stomach, stretch arms forward and put forehead on the floor. Now lift the right arm and left leg simultaneously, hold briefly, lower, then practice on other side. Practice each side five times.

*Practice as long as you enjoy it*

**9.** To recuperate, lie on your side and roll yourself up like a package. Encircle the bent knees with the arms and breathe deeply to give the completely rounded back an opportunity to be filled with air, then stretch out again.

**10.** Resume lying on your back, legs completely stretched out, hands folded behind the neck. Pull yourself slowly up to a sitting position by first lifting the head up and then rolling the torso up. While sitting up, stretch the back thoroughly. Then, keeping legs extended, slide forward by alternately pushing the right and left sides of the pelvis forward.

**11.** Sit with legs extended. Anchor feet under a heavy piece of furniture, clasp the hands behind the head. Keeping the torso taut, lean back several times until you almost reach the floor. Slowly lift torso, reverse and return to sitting position. Repeat three times. While sitting, turn the trunk to the side so that when leaning back the elbow of that same side touches the floor. Sit up again, turn to other side, and repeat.

*Can also be practiced on a stool*

**12.** Sit with crossed legs. Arch the back outward and immediately pull it back in until reaching the hollow of the small of the back. This alternating movement should be done gently and without any friction.

**13.** Still sitting cross-legged, fold the hands in back of neck, stretch and bend the torso as far as possible to one side. Straighten up, then bend to the other side. Repeat 3 times in each direction.

**14.** Start off in a cross-legged position, then switch over to standing on the knees. Place the hands on the hips and slowly sit back on the heels without losing control of the small of the back—i.e., do not fall into the hollow of the small of the back. After practicing three times, turn the torso to the right and then to the left, so that you alternately sit down to the left and right of the feet. Since it is difficult to keep one's balance, only gradually attempt to deepen the movement. Repeat three times toward each side.

*Gradually bend further down*

117

**15.** From the knee position, put your hands down so you are on all fours. Keep the back stretched while raising the right leg and left arm until they are horizontal. Hold, then lower them and repeat with the other side.

**16.** From an all-fours position, stretch both legs back completely until you are in a supported lying position. Hop with one leg into a squatting position while keeping the other leg stretched out. In the interval between these motions, rock lightly up and down twice, then with a hop made while in squatting position, change legs and repeat the exercise five times. Then from the supported lying position take short steps in the direction of the hands until only the fingertips are touching the floor. Slowly bring yourself like a folding pocket knife to a standing position.

*Remember to breathe properly*

**17.** With the arms still raised, make a deep swing downward with the trunk. While doing so, keep the knees elastic and let the head, neck, shoulders and arms swing down with the torso. At the beginning of the movement, the head should fall loosely into the neck before being drawn into the movement by the torso swinging down.

**18.** Let the swinging motion stop by itself, straighten the knees again, and roll up to a standing position. Then bob up and down somewhat so that you alternately put your weight on the ascending foot and none on the descending foot. A gradually increased tempo leads to getting so far off the floor that the movement turns into hopping. Lift the arms, and push the feet down as energetically as if you wanted to reach the ceiling. After approximately one minute, reduce the movement until the simple up-and-down movement of the feet is resumed, then come to a standstill and again lower the arms.

**19.** Bring arms up from the side while inhaling deeply. Holding the palms of the hands down, lower the arms to the side while stretching the torso and slowly exhaling through slightly opened lips. Repeat four times.

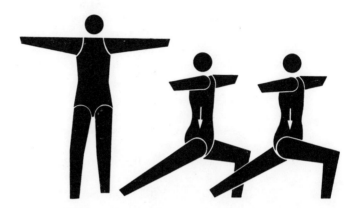

*Arms
laterally
extended
helps
balance*

**20.** Hold the arms shoulder-high, take a slight lunging step
forward. In doing so, bend the front leg enough that the back leg
is almost stretched. Rock up and down as deeply as possible in
this position, keeping the torso upright and stretched. Spring up
and down three times, then jump up and exchange legs. Take at
least ten such deep, bouncing steps.
Rock up and down as deeply as possible in this position, keeping
the torso upright and stretched. Spring up and down three times,
then jump up and exchange legs. Take at least ten such deep,
bouncing steps.
**21.** Swing one leg in a high arch across the side toward the back
and set it down behind the other leg. Repeat using other leg.
**22.** Stand, legs slightly spread apart. Lift the arms along the side
to a vertical position, then lean the torso from one side to the
other without turning upper body.
**23.** After repeating above several times, instead of resuming
vertical position, loosely swing the torso forward and to one
side. Alternate sides and repeat several times.

119

**24.** From the side position of the previous exercise, lift the arms vertically again and stretch all the way to the fingertips. Stretch the body as much as possible, inhale deeply, and while exhaling loosely fall into a deep, crouching position. Repeat two or three times, then lower stretched arms to the sides.

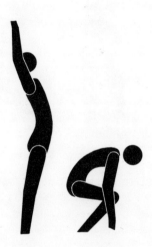

This comprehensive exercise program attempts to include the whole body from head to foot with its muscles, ligaments and joints. Some exercises may be too strenuous and difficult for older and more corpulent persons as, for example, the cross-legged sitting position. Therefore, it should be kept in mind that what applies to exercises directed toward specific problems applies to these exercises as well: exercise should be strenuous but should not cause overexertion. The exercises should be chosen according to what the person is able to do, and gymnastics should be fun. Everyone is encouraged to select exercises they can successfully perform and to set up a program that corresponds to their specific abilities and strength. It is important though that the program include one exercise for each part of the body and for each muscle group.

# Lying, Sitting, Carrying, Lifting and Standing Properly

*The bed must be right for the user*

There is a great and emphatic difference of opinion as to what kind of bed can be considered healthy and good for the discs. In addition, the preference in beds is an extremely individual matter. Apart from a very few general stipulations resulting from the anatomy and physiology of the body, each person must choose a bed that suits him best. It should be kept in mind though that in addition to orthopedic considerations, such factors as circulation and nerves are relevant in the choice of a bed. Many heart patients, for example, cannot lie flat, while some persons suffering from nervous sleep disorders are aided by a slight elevation of the head. Many persons with sensitive stomachs cannot lie completely flat. Persons with liver disease may prefer to lie on their sides with a slight counter-pressure provided by a pillow or roll. Persons with varicose veins may need to be able to have their legs elevated.

*Mechanical considerations of circulation*

Body weight is also a consideration. A heavy person needs a thicker, harder mattress and even a stronger frame than a person of slight or normal stature. Becoming accustomed to a bed with some support can be a nuisance to some; others, after three hours on a firm mattress, may feel their painful hip bones. Sometimes one examines a hotel bed because one has slept exceptionally well on it; at another time it was impossible to fall asleep because of pain in the small of the back. The circumstances and the combination of frame and mattress were different each time. That is why large bedding stores are adopting a policy of letting the customer try different bedding combinations at home, because individual needs can only be determined practically, not theoretically. Some general and important points of view:
- The back should have the possibility of lying flat in order to take the pressure off the discs and to let them convert their metabolism to, suction;

*The right mattress*

- The mattress should have a wool covering to absorb moisture. The best mattress material remains horsehair, but unfortunately it is very expensive;
- The frame should be firm but resilient, and there should be a possibility of raising the head and foot of the bed;
- The mattress should be all of one piece, not made up of two or

121

three pieces;
• The mattress should correspond in thickness and firmness to body weight. Bed covers should be light and airy.

One important element of good sleep should not be overlooked: the ability to tune things out and relax, or emotional stability. A person under emotional stress will still sleep fitfully in his orthopedically irreproachable bed, whereas someone else may get a good night's sleep even on straw.

*Sitting properly.* The assertion that to sit for longer than one hour is actually unhealthy is a valid starting point for considering all problems related to sitting. Yet, in view of the many responsibilities faced by everyone during the course of a day, it is difficult or impossible to heed such a precept. The compression of the spinal column that results from sitting is the source of the greatest pressure on the spinal column and particularly on the discs. Their regenerative capacity is consequently responsive to traction *(see p. 43)*. These basic facts, in any case, provide an orientation for considering the problems resulting from sitting and for deciding which factors might make sitting healthier, or at least physiologically more sound.

*Sitting— #1 stress factor for discs*

One main reason that sitting places a stress on the spinal column is that a sitting position eliminates its physiological curves. For the curves are what give the spinal column its elasticity, and it is the curves that can change a rigid rod subject to hard jolts into a subtle elastic spinal column capable of distributing the pressure to which it is subject. As these curves build on one another and interact, it is primarily important in sitting that the first curvature—i.e., that the slightly concave arching in the lumbar vertebral column (lumbar lordosis) be pronounced and capable of influencing the other curves.

*Loss of elasticity*

This first adjustment of the pelvis is important for the back while in a sitting position. The cup-shaped design of seating for the Munich Olympics took this particular physiological detail into consideration. Although there were no backs to the seating, a slight protrusion along the back edge of the seat positioned the pelvis up and forward, which is characteristic of good seating. The functional design of the Olympic seating illustrates that a minimum of proper support for the back in the right place is often more effective than a comfortable chair with a back whose curves are wrongly placed.

The most important part of a chair is therefore the lower part

of the chair back—i.e., the part on ladder-back chairs so popular
for use at the dining table that regrettably consists of a slat or of
open space. However much such designs may fit in with the
style of other surrounding furniture, they are not conceived to fit
the back or to meet its needs.

There are now sensible accessories for car and office seating
that make adjustments possible both for the small of the back
and for the height of the back. Several large firms have created
well-planned workplaces by the use of work surfaces high
enough to be used while standing or while sitting on an adjustable
stool. Such measures to a large extent comply both with the
needs of work and of the back.

*Standing* is primarily tiring for the small of the back. It also
strains the feet, the legs, and the circulation. If there is enough
space to allow some movement while standing, the strain is
significantly diminished. The spinal column should also periodi-
cally be loosened up by various movements of the pelvis,
especially in the small of the back.

*Standing
and shoes*

Comfortable shoes that are roomy enough for the toes to be
curled up and moved about should be worn. Under certain
circumstances, a change of shoes should be made frequently. A
change of heel height also changes back strain. Then, too, it may
be desirable to wear shoes that can easily be slipped off to give
the feet a chance to recuperate.

Several questions repeatedly posed concerning shoes are:
what is the relationship between back pain and shoes? Which
height heel is best? Which type shoe is best? Since all these
questions are much subject to the dictates of fashion, anyone
who likes comfortable shoes runs the danger of looking
ridiculous. Designs conceived for reasons of health have not yet
proved to be a fashion success, and if they were to become a
success, fashion would promptly declare them boring and
uninteresting. Although the dictates of fashion may crave
change, health factors know no season, so the best available
advice is to change shoes frequently, since each change of heel
height changes the static relationships and distributes pressures
anew. Everything is permitted, from going barefoot at home and

*Tensing
muscles
helps
circulation*

in the garden to wearing flat or high heels as long as the shoes
are changed often.

Every movement of the feet and legs while standing reduces
strain on the circulation. Standing briefly on the toes, for

123

example, tenses the entire leg musculature, thereby promoting the return of venous blood and impeding blood from "sinking" into the legs. By vigorously flexing the foot while keeping the leg stretched, the calf muscle is stretched and its circulation is improved. By briefly and energetically bending the knee toward the back, the knee joint is exercised and the upper thigh musculature is stretched.

Workplaces too cramped to permit periodic movement, where there is little standing room, or where even perching on the edge of a high stool is not permitted certainly reflect no regard for health. As an expression of social policy, they are indefensible, particularly considering the immense annual cost of absences due to back aches and disc problems.

*Careful when lifting and twisting simultaneously*

*Lifting and carrying* objects place still another strain on the body. Lifting while simultaneously turning or bending the torso is the most dangerous combination of exertion. It often occurs while unloading the trunk of a car. Great strain is placed on the back if one lifts a heavy load and turns while the back is bent, because from this position the greatest amount of strength is needed for lifting the weight at some distance from the body, and the small of the back has to function as a lever. If a heavy load can only be lifted in the manner just described, any attempt to lift it unassisted should be avoided if at all possible, even if this necessitates senselessly transporting a case of beer all over town during the day in order to wait for help in unloading it in the evening.

As every professional weightlifter knows, objects to be lifted from the floor should be picked up while crouching down and should be lifted and carried very close to the body.

By using a little imagination, it is usually possible to distribute the weight of many objects between both hands. Often what may be needed is simply a second shopping bag or two suitcases instead of one, a minor but very worthwhile investment.

An almost insolvable problem in terms of the proper technique of carrying about weight is posed by children's schoolbags. Their weight, even if carried on the children's backs, is a health liability, and would even overtax adults. Schools, parents, and teachers should find possibilities of relieving children, even ten-year-olds, of the burden of dragging whole libraries back and forth between school and home.

The combination of simultaneously exerting strength and

124

twisting the body is also necessary in tennis and golf, so persons predisposed toward disc problems, sciatica, and lumbago should choose their sports activities carefully. Playing tennis or golf after an interval of not having engaged in these sports can frequently result in an attack of lumbago. Such an attack can also occur while getting out of a low sports car after a long ride.

# The Roles of Therapist—Patient

What can the therapist do?

On the basis of some knowledge about the context of back pain, it may be well to recall once again the various possibilities of therapy and prevention:

*Backaches*
*as a symp-*
*tom of*
*disturbance*

If pain exists, a doctor must first be consulted to establish the cause and make a differential diagnosis. Keep in mind that back pain is not a disease but is a symptom of a disturbance.

If necessary, medication should be used to alleviate the pain. Further treatment involving medication should be under the supervision of a doctor.

It is possible that chiropractic manipulation may be effective in pushing back into a place a small dislocated intervertebral joint and in relieving pain. The success of chiropractic treatment may not be lasting and usually should be supplemented by massage and gymnastics.

Several measures that may be helpful in reducing pain include appropriate positioning of the patient, stretching of the spinal column by means of traction apparatus, and the use of heat. Often it is necessary to find out which form of heat is most effective—whether to use hot, wet applications or radiation therapy, using different wavelengths ranging from infrared or short wave or even the use of x-ray treatment in rare cases.

*Fibrous*
*tissue*
*massage*

For acute stages of pain, carefully chosen gymnastic exercises, especially certain tensing and pulling exercises, bring relief. Certain types of massage are also effective. Fibrous tissue massage produces the greatest stimulation to circulation by widening the capillaries and small arteries in the fibrous tissues by means of a stretching stimulus, which in turn triggers a reflex in the blood vessels. The warming effect even in the tissues is therefore immense; since it exerts less pull on the musculature than muscle massage, it is particularly effective for acute pain.

The goal of muscle massage is to stimulate circulation and to

125

*Muscle massage*

loosen up the muscles by techniques of stretching and by kneading and pressing the myogelosis.

Therapeutically controlled exercises done in water offer the relief of weightlessness, which can release severe muscle cramps. The water must be warm enough, however, to avoid heightening muscle tension. The temperature threshold is approximately 82° F.

# Keeping Your Back Working Properly

*Recognizing changes early*

What is important is to observe and detect changes early, to relieve tension, and to mobilize stiffness. More accurately, the goal is to try to keep muscles functional, the spinal column flexible, and the discs elastic.

The following is a summary of ideas and advice concerning self-help:
• Maintain the functioning ability of your back muscles by using them often.
• Ensure good muscle circulation by alternately tensing and relaxing them frequently.
• Strengthen your back musculature by engaging in a carefully considered exercise program.
• Keep your chest elastic by repeatedly stretching the ligaments and joints.
• Give your discs some relief by using them more frequently in the course of the day in the "pull" position.
• Keep your spinal column flexible through the use of mobilizing exercises.
• Try to learn to relax through the help of yoga, gymnastics, or autogenic training.
• Try, if it is necessary and possible, to improve conditions where you work. Often even a minor change such as using a different chair, using a foot rest, or support for the back in the proper spot can bring perceptible relief.
• Engage in playful sports activity that does not involve ambition or stress the level of accomplishment.
• Keep in mind the particular problem involved with speed, its

126

effect on the back muscles, and the difficulty of adjusting to an alien tempo.

• Consider yourself first in setting the rhythm of your life.

• Try whenever possible to stimulate your breathing mechanism, and make certain that you get plenty of fresh air during the day and before sleeping.

• Stimulate circulation by walking briskly. Strolling will not accomplish this purpose.

• Condition yourself by training your capacity that the frame and mattress are right for your body.

• Control your weight. Stay within the norm, because each pound of overweight is a burden on your discs.

• Above all, remember that back pains often have an emotional basis. Keep in mind that, just as psychological burdens can be redistributed, tolerance can be learned. Physical and emotional reserves are not inexhaustible.

It is reassuring to know that not all back pain is permanent and that an interval in one's life marred by back pain can be followed by a completely pain-free period.

*Self-healing is possible* Remember, too, that there is a kind of self-healing, even for the area of the back.

• And, finally, realize that good health is not merely the absence of disease. An important factor in man's wellbeing consists in his ability to learn to live with his particular physical propensities and limitations.